The Psychological Immune System
A New Look At Protection and Survival

Herman Kagan, Ph.D.

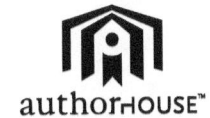

authorHOUSE™

1663 LIBERTY DRIVE, SUITE 200
BLOOMINGTON, INDIANA 47403
(800) 839-8640
WWW.AUTHORHOUSE.COM

First published by AuthorHouse 12/15/05

ISBN: 1-4208-9005-0 (sc)
ISBN: 1-4208-9004-2 (eb)

Library of Congress Control Number: 2005908995

Printed in the United States of America

Bloomington, Indiana

This book is printed on acid-free paper.

PREFACE

Today, psychology is an enormous force-both scientifically and clinically- in the ongoing effort to understand the sources of human behavior. As biology and medicine make rapid advances in the physical aspects of behavior, psychology has been greatly challenged to match these advances with its own productivity utilizing the scientific method. Sigmund Freud remarked that he looked forward to the day when his concepts and ideas would receive substantiation from neurologists who would be able to report the specific areas of the brain wherein ego, superego and id reside.

This thrust to connect what is known about the physiology of the body with the psychological constructs of modern day, may be the purpose behind Dr. Herman Kagan's remarkable book, "The Psychological Immune System." It is a ground-breaking effort to tie together the biological immune system functioning, and its logical counterpart in the human psyche. It is particularly interesting to see this within an evolutionary framework. It is one of the concepts that is so logical one might sit back and say, "Of course, why didn't I think of that."

Perhaps anticipating skepticism from the rowdy world of scientific controversy, Dr. Kagan builds his case for the Psychological Immune System brick-by-brick, drawing us in with personal anecdotes, supporting his structure with a wide-ranging review of the literature on pertinent anthropological studies, biology and genetic findings, animal and human development and a host of other fascinating ideas. He reminds us of the empirical support for theories of self-image, evolution, and the development of societies. He organizes this knowledge in a compelling way that reads easily and makes us more open to his interesting inferences.

It is one thesis of Dr. Kagan's book that the idea of a psychological immune system extend beyond the individual and has application to groups, organizations and even nations. He has taken some pains to develop an initial system of weighting key features and principles of his theoretical model to facilitate evaluation of a given human situation.

It is a book likely to stir the emotions and the brain in roughly equal measures. I perceive it as a pioneering, serious effort to remind us of the human condition under which all of us try to do our best in the struggle to fulfill our ambitions and protect our loved ones under increasing complex social conditions.

Richard Reinhart, Ph.D.
Ventura, California

ACKNOWLEDGMENTS

Writing a book requires almost endless motivation, patience, and endurance. Many times one has to push oneself to keep going when ideas and selection of material are not flowing freely. It can be both a challenging and humbling experience. Thus, it is extremely beneficial to have an ongoing source of inspiration and people who provide positive incentives.

From the beginning my inspiration for writing this book came from my grandchildren, Jacob and Sarah, whom I dearly love. This love kindled the desire to leave them with things I've learned during my journey in this world, as a clinical psychologist, father, and grandfather. Something they could use when they're grown, on their own, have their own families, and want to pass on what they've learned.

While the initial inspiration came from my grandchildren, it soon became obvious to me that my desire to leave behind some of my knowledge extended to other family members, as well, like Hanky, Nicky, Briana, Sharon, Hailie and Mailani. From there, my desire became more and more encompassing to include all potential parents and teachers as well as the parents and teachers who are currently active. After I got started, the belief that I had something to offer was the fuel that kept my engine running even when I sputtered along.

This belief was thankfully reinforced by people who were willing to read some of the chapters as they were being written or listen to tapes I recorded about the book and give me feedback about their reaction to the idea of a psychological immune system, their understanding of the contents, and questions that came to mind. I was fortunate to get a diverse group of people. First, there were members of my family : my wife, Verna, an attorney who manages a pro bono program for the county bar association, my daughter Batya, who has a degree in environmental science, and my cousin, Shana Blumenthal, who has a bachelors degree in psychology and works for Children's Protective Services. Then there were my professional colleagues and friends consisting of Virginia Johnson, a college instructor for business issues , Sonya Gerlach, a licensed clinical social worker in private practice; Dr. Ron Bale, a licensed psychologist in private practice who also helps in the training of UCLA medical residents; Dr. Roger Coger, a licensed psychologist in private practice; Dr. Gil McFarlane, a licensed psychologist employed by Ventura County with an expertise in neuropsychology, and Dr. Richard Reinhart, a licensed psychologist in private practice and formally Chief Psychologist in the Ventura County Mental Health Department. Last, but not least, were my neighbors Robert Barnett, a deputy sheriff and Carrie Burton, an elementary school teacher, each of whom are dedicated and successful parents. Everyone mentioned provided valuable critiques that made me think and rethink regarding the book's contents and the audience that might benefit from the book. They all deserve my heartfelt thanks.

I would also like to extend my appreciation to Eric Larsen of Studio e Books who took on the task of editing my manuscript and making it more grammatically correct, more condensed, and much more readable.

It wouldn't be fair to close out the acknowledgments without mentioning and extending my deepest appreciation to all the children and families who gave me the opportunity to know and interact with them and from whom many of the ideas of the book were generated. A special thanks belongs to the Vargas family, of whom my daughter-in-law, Lupe, is a member, for demonstrating so clearly the importance of identity in family cohesiveness.

TABLE OF CONTENTS

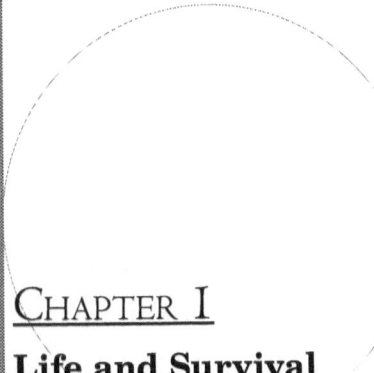

CHAPTER I

Life and Survival
Built-In Mechanisms and Strategies

ATTENDING TO OUR EMOTIONS

The night ended like many others. After drinking beer, singing, dancing, and soaking in the music and atmosphere of the German beer hall, we were reminded by the clock of our curfew and the need to return to the army base and our barracks. So the six of us left the beer hall, piled into the big black 1950 Buick that one of the lucky soldiers owned, and headed back to the 7th Army headquarters on the outskirts of Stuttgart, Germany. We were joking, laughing, and having a raucous good time driving along one of the streets in Stuttgart, and then suddenly we heard the scraping of metal and were startled for a moment before we realized that we had sideswiped a parked car. Our driver just kept on going, turning off his lights so the black car would mingle with the darkness of

1

the night in case a witness was at hand. The momentary anxiety produced even more laughter, like that of kids running from a produce stand after knocking over some vegetables.

My own beer-influenced brain raced through several different feelings. The macho-male-military part of me was enjoying the excitement. But my cautious-vulnerable side was worried about riding in a car that was being driven rather recklessly, while my moral sense triggered thoughts of stopping and trying to find the owner of the car we had just hit. In the end, the reinforcement of the all-male company having a good time won out, so I joined in the laughter and stimulation of the moment all the way back to the base where I bid all my army buddies a good night.

Throughout the week, my mind replayed that evening many times over, and I still felt the emotional tug-of-war between the conflicting emotions circulating through my brain. The thrill of going to town with a bunch of other guys; the excitement of the recklessness and escape artistry of the driver; the concern for my safety, and the shame for allowing the carefree part of my personality to take control of my behavior during the ride back to the base.

The issue was not totally settled when the next weekend came and the same five soldiers came by in the black Buick and offered me a ride downtown. Because I showed a little hesitation, the group urged a little harder. When pushed to the wall, however, my anxiety took over and I made an excuse and told them that I would take a rain check. So they drove off without me and I was left with the feeling that the "chicken" part of me had somehow spoken more loudly than the adventurous and macho part.

When you think about it, it is amazing that the simple decision of whether or not to go for a ride in a car can be so complicated. There are issues of safety , pleasure, peer acceptance, self-image, and moral judgment, each has its own emotional component wiggling its way into awareness. Yet somehow the mixture of all these components is juggled, and a decision comes forth. We don't know, usually, whether the decision is a "good" or "bad" one until the consequences of our judgment are played out and evaluated later on.

If the group of guys had come upon me the next day and told me of the wonderful time they had had and the sensuous ladies they had met, I would have chided myself for being so cautious and "uptight." If they had told me they had gotten into an argument with some of the patrons of the beer hall and could have used an extra body, I would have felt bad about letting the group down. If they had come back and told me about getting into a discussion about the war and how the German patrons had made excuses for their behavior, I would have felt sad for missing the opportunity to voice my own opinion.

As it was however, the group didn't meet me the next day, or any other day, because they never made it back to the base. The Buick was totaled when the driver crashed into a concrete pillar while negotiating a turn onto the highway. All five soldiers were killed! The company commander had the wrecked car hauled onto the base to show the rest of us the result of drinking and driving. This created quite a bit of resentment among the rank-and-file soldiers, who pointed to the eleven o'clock curfew as the real culprit. For me it was a sobering reminder of how crucial each of our decisions can be and proved that we never know when our lives hang in the balance. It is a lesson I have never forgotten and it taught me much greater respect for my anxiety.

While decision-making at the psychological level requires us to juggle many different considerations- such as our life and physical well-being, our social status, our family connections, and our moral judgments-we cannot make good decisions without our emotions. If it wasn't for the arousal of my feeling of apprehension and allowing that feeling to guide my decision, I would have been dead at the ripe- young age of twenty-four, a scary and sobering thought.

That we need our emotions to make good decisions about our future is underscored by studies done by Damasio[1] and others who have described the disastrous consequences of individuals who have lost their emotional faculties due to brain damage, even though their cognitive, intellectual and memory capabilities remained intact. It seems we comprehend life's events through their emotional impact on us, and our emotions act as warning signals for the dangers we encounter. This parallels the signals pain and discomfort send regarding injuries to our body. In fact, individuals who are born without the sense of pain rarely live beyond age thirty, as pain stops us from re-exposing our injured body to further trauma.[2]

While it is true that too much emotion can be detrimental to one's judgment and decision-making, it is still important to realize that emotions allow us to weigh complex perceptions, interactions, and situations and come up with a plan of action that protects, preserves, and enhances important aspects of ourselves and our lives.

The phenomenon of an essential trait becoming detrimental when it is too intense, too concentrated, too frequent or out of control can be found throughout nature. For example, too much pain, too much fever, too much growth, too much speed, too much heat, and a too intense immune reaction can all be detrimental. However, just the opposite is also true: too little pain, too little growth, too little speed, too little heat, and a too subdued immune reaction are also detrimental. It is important to keep in mind that because something can be detrimental at times, this doesn't detract from its importance. This certainly applies to pain and emotion which help us survive.

SURVIVAL MECHANISMS

Evolution has provided us humans with tools that enable us to survive, just as it has provided other life forms with tools that enable them to survive. In many cases, our survival mechanisms are very similar. That is why scientists can study the immune systems of rats and chimpanzees and relate the findings to our own immune system. That is why scientists can study and manipulate DNA in the cells of bacteria and yeast and apply the findings to our own DNA. That is why human genes can be inserted into the DNA of bacteria, yeast, and rats and have our genes replicated.[3]

It appears that survival is built into all life forms, from one-celled organisms to human beings. This means both adapting to environmental conditions and developing a reproductive rate greater than the death rate. If this were not the case, how could one explain the unbroken chain of life over 3 1/2 billion years even though many species have vanished. How could one explain the adaptations of organisms to such extreme environments as hydrothermal vents of boiling water under the oceans, scalding thermal pools in Yellowstone National Park, lakes so alkaline they can burn human flesh, rocks so deep below the surface of the earth that the pressure can crush bones and microbes that can thrive on organic solvents such as kerosene and benzene that are toxic to other life forms.[4, 5]

Certainly natural selection is at work as many individual organisms and species succumb before they can adapt and reproduce. However, were it not for the built-in life-sustaining processes of cells and their adaptability via gene mutations, natural selection would never have the opportunity to work.

Take the single-cell bacteria, for example. When they encounter a reduced food supply, what do they do? The common soil bacterium, *Bacillus sphaericus*, divides unevenly, forming a larger mother cell and a smaller daughter cell which is engulfed by the mother cell. The daughter cell is then nurtured by the mother cell, which uses its energy to stitch together a protein coat for the daughter cell. The mother cell then bursts open, dies, and releases the protein-coated daughter cell which is called a spore. The spore can survive for years until a suitable food supply is available, at which time the spore returns to its original bacterial state.

The myxobacteria, another soil-dwelling species, forms a fruiting body with up to 100,000 individual bacteria that join together to form a stalk topped by one or more small spore balls filled with bacteria. The spores, which make up about 10 to 20 percent of the fruiting body, survive, while the other 80 to 90,000 cells that make up the stalk break open and die. The strategy of individuals dying for the preservation of the group is one that has been built into many different species. How decisions are made about which individuals are to live and which are to die is still a mystery to scientists.

Microbiologist James Shapiro of the University of Chicago, who has worked with Escherichia coli, the common gut bacteria, believes that an E. coli colony is a highly organized structure and that its members can communicate with each other by some means. Thus, when a colony is attacked by a type of virus known as a bacteriophage, a protective layer of cells forms which takes the brunt of the attack and whose cells are destroyed while the cells beneath it survive. Shapiro believes that E. coli uses the same strategy to protect itself from other agents as well, such as antibiotics and disinfectants.[6] And other bacteria, like Caulobacter crescentus, feed off the nutrients released by their dead siblings.[7]

These interactive survival strategies are matched by similar mechanisms that have evolved for plants. For example, Dischidia major, a plant in the Malaysian part of Borneo, is an epiphyte, a plant that lacks soil-penetrating roots and instead wraps itself around other plants that it needs for support. These plants rely on raindrops and moisture in the air for their few nutrient supplies. But Dischidia also provides a home for ants in its sac-shaped leaves. In return, the plant uses ant breath as a source of carbon dioxide and ant debris as a source of nitrogen.[8]

Trees produce resin to cover their injuries and protect themselves from infection. Many plants produce potent chemicals that help protect them from insects and other enemies. Tomato plants, for example, produce the allelochemicals chlorgenic acid, rutin, and tomatine, which are natural anti-insect compounds that slow insect development and make invasive insects more vulnerable to predators. Likewise, oak buds and acorns are loaded with nutrients, but potential consumers have to be careful about eating them raw because they are loaded with tannins and alkaloids, which are toxic to animals. Early Europeans who ate unprocessed acorns died even sooner than their starving companions. In fact, plants that defend themselves chemically against herbivores have created weapons and defenses of enormous power and diversity, including digitalis, opioids, caffeine, and cocaine.[9]

Multicellular animals have developed many different survival mechanisms. Bees, for example, live in large colonies and have workers who protect their hives by recognizing and attacking intruders. Stinging protects bees from most intruders, but not from the giant Japanese hornets, which are three times the size of the European honeybees imported to Japan about 120 years ago. A single hornet can kill up to forty bees a minute with its powerful jaws, and a group of about twenty hornets can wipe out an entire colony of

30,000 bees in about three hours. So what do the bees do? When a hornet enters the hive some 500 workers surround it in a dense ball and vibrate their wings until the temperature inside the bee ball goes up to 116° Fahrenheit. Hornets die at 114° whereas bees can tolerate temperatures up to 122 degrees. After about fifteen minutes of baking, the hornet dies, according to entomologist Masato Ono of Tamagawa University in Tokyo.[10] Isn't nature remarkable!

Insects have exoskeletons to protect them from being punctured, and beetles have the toughest armor of all. To stick a pin through some beetles for scientific mounting, a hammer is required. Some insects use chemical warfare to protect themselves. The European bombardier beetle, for example, fires a boiling hot jet of noxious chemicals at attackers in a series of high speed pulses.[11]

In addition to armor and chemicals to protect them from environmental hazards, insects use camouflage, disguises, brightly colored warnings, mimicry, playing dead, and high-frequency sound that can jam the sonar of bats. They seem to use the techniques of modern armies-or perhaps it's the other way around. There are also complicated systems of communication among insects, with bees able to inform their hive mates where to locate distant food sources via their circle-and-waggle dance. Barbara Shipman, a mathematician at the University of Rochester, found that the bee's dance conforms to the mathematical equations that describe the geometrical patterns of quarks-the tiny particles that are the building blocks of protons and neutrons. She believes the relationship between the bee's dance and the behavior of quarks is no mere coincidence. She suspects that the bees are somehow sensitive to what's going on in the quantum world of quarks.[12] If she can prove this, there is surely a Nobel prize waiting for her.

THE EMERGENCE OF THE IMMUNE SYSTEM

Using vision, hearing, and a smell sense, insects have sophisticated ways of finding food, to which any human can attest when out for a walk, a picnic, or a backyard barbecue. Crawling, walking, or flying, they seem to hone in on food sources and they don't seem to mind if the food is dead or alive, ingested or excreted. While they help clean up the mess on our planet, they also carry many diseases, some of which can threaten our survival.

Mosquitoes, for example, can transmit through their bite viruses and other pathogens that produce dengue, hemorrhagic fever, yellow fever, and malaria, to name but a few. Ticks carry pathogens that produce Colorado tick fever, Rocky Mountain spotted fever, and Lyme disease. Fleas, mites, flies, and other creatures carry the additional disorders of typhus, sleeping sickness, Chagas' disease and rickettsial diseases.[13] With all these pathogens and more running around the earth, our survival depends on a system of defense against their onslaught, and indeed we have such defenses, courtesy of evolution.

The immune system as we know it, with its ability to provide rapid antibody responses, originated in warm-blooded vertebrates such as birds and mammals and can be traced back to the Triassic period, some 230 million years ago.[14, 15] The forerunners of the immune system, however, go back to one celled animals, like the amoeba, which feed by recognizing non-self substances and rejecting or ingesting them. This trait, which was and still is needed for self-preservation, became a characteristic of all multicellular organisms. It can be seen in the sponges, which are commonly regarded as the most primitive of present-day animals. For example, interfacial fusion (uniting together) can occur between sponges from the same colony, but members of different colonies reject each other.[16]

The human immune system relies on its ability to distinguish between self and non-self cells and protein for effective functioning. In fact, our immune system can be thought of as a specialized system that has evolved to protect and preserve our life and physical well-being from invasion by foreign substances, especially microorganisms. Once inside us, microorganisms can take over or destroy our cells and disrupt processes essential to our survival. In this way , our immune system can also be thought of as an extension of the survival mechanisms built into all life forms. It has been selected by the evolutionary process because it helps us preserve and protect our bodies from destructive pathogens and gives us more time to reproduce before we die. In essence, the immune system helps us come to grips with a world teeming with microorganisms.

It has been estimated, for example, that we carry around a concentration of at least 10,000 microorganisms per square centimeter of our skin, and that scrapings from our teeth and gums may contain millions of microorganisms, just as does our saliva. We also excrete trillions of organisms from our intestines on a daily basis.[17]

Thus our immune system has quite a task assigned to it. By recognizing which proteins and cells are part of the body and which are not, it takes an important first step in doing its job. By attacking and destroying that which does not belong to the body, it provides protection to the body. However, this protection also makes it difficult to transplant foreign or donor tissue and organs. By recognizing specific pathogens that have attacked the body and maintaining a memory of them via memory cells, the immune system can more rapidly dispose of the same pathogens when it encounters them again. The use of vaccines takes advantage of this trait and the ability of the immune system to build up an antibody and T-cell response to the same pathogen to which the vaccine exposed us.

It seems, then, that speed of response is an important factor for survival, both on the part of an animal being attacked by a predator and an animal being attacked by microorganisms. One can easily see why evolution has selected for this trait and why our immune system makes such prominent use of it in our war with pathogens. But the recognition of a non-self substance only gets the ball rolling, so to speak. Next, the nonspecific or innate component of the immune system-which makes use of phagocytosis, toxic chemicals, and enzymes-take on pathogens that enter the body and attempts to neutralize or destroy them. However, if the pathogens evade the nonspecific or innate component of the system, they are met by the specific or acquired component of the system. Some of the millions of different antibodies that are produced by our white blood cells, of the B-cell variety, find a fit with the antigens of the invader. Once this occurs, clones of that particular antibody are manufactured by B-cells that enlarge into plasma cells. These antibodies can overwhelm and destroy the invading pathogens. The newly cloned antibodies result from antigen exposure, and that is the reason scientists speak of the "acquired" component of the immune system.[18]

When the immune system is functioning efficiently, it relies on, (1) its ability to discriminate between self and non self substances; (2) its ability to mount a nonspecific or generalized attack against the invader; (3) its ability to identify the specific antigen of the invading pathogen; (4) its ability to mount a specific attack against the invader; (5) its ability to remember that antigen ; (6) its ability to mount a much faster and more concentrated antibody or T-cell response to the same antigen in the future; (7) its ability to use a homeostatic process to regulate the intensity and duration of the response to the invader and to cease responding once the invading pathogen has been disposed of.[19]

Many of these same processes are also used by animals in trying to avoid predators. They too must identify the predator, show versatility in avoiding and handling an attack, prepare for a faster response the second time around, and calm down once the predator is no longer around. The homeostatic process, which controls the ebb and flow of energy and productivity, is crucial to sustaining the life and well-being of organisms from one-celled to us humans. It monitors the buildup and outpouring of energy and assures that there is a return to a less active state in which energy can be renewed and conserved. An ultrahigh energy level or state of enhanced activation that is maintained over a long period of time can be too draining and can be detrimental to life and physical well-being. This can be seen when we are under stress for too long a period and our adrenal glands respond by secreting too much cortisol, which can lead to organ and brain damage.[20]

IMMUNE SYSTEM MALFUNCTIONS

Although our immune system protects us from disease-causing organisms most of the time, there are also instances in which it fails to rise to the occasion or overdoes itself. The results can include the flare-up of opportunistic diseases, tissue damage, toxic reactions, and autoimmune reactions. The immune system's under reaction to various antigens is known as immunodeficiency. This can have a genetic base, or it can be acquired as a result of disease. The best known is acquired immune deficiency syndrome (AIDS), with resulting opportunistic infections from protozoa, bacteria, and fungi.[21]

The most familiar overreaction to non-threatening antigens is an allergic disorder. The most common allergic disorders are the reactions to poison ivy and poison oak. More dangerous, but more rare, are overreactive responses to insect stings and penicillin injections, resulting in shock and airway obstruction. Similarly, overproduction of plasma cells, which produce antibodies, can cause tumors in bone marrow or the infiltration of tissue and organs with insoluble protein fibrils.[22]

In autoimmune reactions, the body's own cells and proteins are treated as though they were foreign antigens and are attacked by the immune system. Sometimes a specific organ, such as the thyroid gland or pancreas, is the target of an autoimmune attack and at other times the attack is nonspecific. Rheumatoid arthritis, insulin-dependent diabetes mellitus, hemolytic anemia, and multiple sclerosis are diseases that are believed to result from autoimmune reactions.[23] Of the estimated 8.5 million people in the United States who suffer from an autoimmune disorder, almost 75 percent are female. Scientists are still trying to determine whether sex hormones influence or even drive the genes that are associated with autoimmunity.[24]

As stated earlier, the immune system can be seen as a special extension of the survival mechanisms that are built into all of life. As a result, the principles and processes that guide the mechanisms of the immune system and other life forms parallel each other and overlap. Among these overlapping principles and processes are the following: (1) organisms must have some way of discriminating between themselves and other substances or organisms in their environment; (2) organisms must have some scheme or process to avoid or exclude the things that can be harmful to them; (3) organisms must have some way to neutralize or destroy harmful invaders; (4) organisms must have some way to regulate their response to an invasion and to shut down the response once the invader has been neutralized or destroyed; and (5) organisms must have some way of learning from past encounters so they can be more efficient in the future. These principles also apply to organisms that form groups, colonies and societies.

Bacteria, ants, bees, lions, chimpanzees, and humans are all watchful for intruders who do not belong to their colony, hive, group, pride or social organization. Bacteria have antigens and recognition sites, ants have soldiers, bees have workers, lions have adult pride members, chimpanzees have the alpha and beta coalition, and humans have all of these and more, including border guards and the Immigration and Naturalization Service. When invaded, bacteria have toxins, ants have pincers and armor coating, bees have stingers, lions have claws and teeth, chimpanzees have trees, teeth and strong arms, and humans have everything from guns to tanks to nerve gas. When the invader is vanquished, all of these animals have sensory organs that provide input and feedback that tell them to stop defending themselves and start attending to any injuries that may have resulted. By means of mutation in bacteria; chemical and physical signals between and within insects; visual, auditory, and olfactory among the higher mammals; and memory of trivia and detail among humans, all learn from past encounters-or they wouldn't be around anymore.

THE PSYCHOLOGICAL IMMUNE SYSTEM: OUR PROGRAM FOR SURVIVAL

In essence, then, like all other animals we have been programmed to survive. Like all primates, we have developed versatility in coping with new environments, new situations, predators, and social challenges. Like them we use hiding, flight, scolding and mobbing, threatening, and attacking types of behavior.[25] Although chimpanzees share some tool-making skills with us humans, we have become tool-makers and technologists par excellence. The use of stone technology dates back some 2.4 million years, and the use of technology seems to have evolved in parallel with the growth of our brains and complex societies,[26] but most probably our technological skills go back even further, to our bipedal ancestors of some 4 million years ago, and possibly longer.

The book *From Lucy To Language*, by Donald Johanson and Blake Edgar, states that stone tools "first appear in the geological record about 2.5 million years ago, at least 1.5 million years after our ancestors became bipedal. Hence the connection between big brains, tool use, and bipedalism has been effectively uncoupled."[27] However, the fact that stone tools have been preserved over the years does not mean that branches from trees and wood of all kind were not used as tools and weapons long before stone became the material of choice for our ancestors. Unfortunately, wood does not preserve well, so stone has been used by paleoanthropologists as the marker for the beginning of tool-making. We apparently need to unearth an australopithecine skeleton whose bony hand is clutching a long piece of petrified wood, with animal remains nearby.

While our tool-making and higher technology have helped us survive in a multitude of environments ranging from sweltering to freezing, mountainous to flatland, wet to dry, and forested to desert, they have also enabled us to destroy other species of animals and plants we have encountered-as well as other humans. Sometimes it seems that we are on a course of self-destruction instead of self-preservation. Yet, despite our destructive behavior we are still reproducing faster than we are dying, and as a result the earth is now host to a human population of over 6 billion members. At least 3,500 different cultural groups make up this population.[28] Perhaps the only environment on earth in which humans have not been able to make their home is underwater, and, who knows, we may overcome that obstacle in the near future.

If we look at how our genetically programmed attempt to survive manifests itself in individuals, within families, within social groups and within nations, we see a multitude of behaviors, programs, processes, and institutions. All have the goal of protecting, preserving, and enhancing our lives and physical well-being as well as the lives and physical well-being of those we love, care about, or with whom we have a sense of belonging. We, like the ancestors of our Homo line, make the utmost use of our symbolic abilities and the creativity that goes hand in hand with these abilities.

Homo habilis, who lived some 2 million years ago, is credited as the first stone-tool-maker and is believed to have used his tools to skin and butcher animals. This allowed him to take the meat to a safe place, away from other predators. However, there is still debate whether Homo habilis was a hunter or just a scavanger.[29] Then, in Africa about 1.4 million years ago, new tools came into use. Hand axes, cleavers, and picks complemented the old tools made by chipping flakes from stones. Homo erectus is credited with this new technology, in which intentional shaping of stones was practiced.[30]

In the evolutionary progression from Homo habilis and Homo erectus to Homo sapiens-modern humans- the sophistication of tools also evolved. Whereas Homo erectus had hand axes, Homo sapiens developed spears, then bows and arrows and guns of all kinds. Whereas Homo erectus knew the use of fire and lived in caves to protect himself, Homo sapiens developed hearths that incorporated draft channels and warming stones for more efficient cooking, and moved out of his caves and erected man-made shelters some 40,000 years ago. Post holes, mammoth bones, and blocks of limestone were commonly used as support for these shelters. A winter camp discovered in Mezhirich, Russia, was found to contain at least five bone houses dating back some 14,000 to 18,000 years. One of the houses had been built with 385 mammoth bones. A semicircle of skulls, topped by a second layer of skulls, pelvises, and scapulae, formed the inner wall, and ninety five mandibles fortified the outer wall.[31]

In modern societies we too depend on shelter, tools, and fire for survival. We keep out or let in the sun and wind. We make use of fire to warm our shelters or air conditioning to cool them. We use tools to build and repair our shelters and weapons to destroy them. We defend our homes, our cities, and our nations with weaponry of all kinds, and use our weapons to intimidate others into conforming with our wishes, whether it be during a criminal act, a police action, or a national action such as has recently taken place in Yugoslavia, Afghanistan, and Iraq. Our weapons, which are manifestations of our survival needs driving our creative powers, have brought humankind to the brink of destruction. Just as the biological immune system can use its awesome powers to destroy its own body, so the survival programs of our psychological immune system, using the awesome powers of technology, can be mis-directed to destroy humanity. Suffice it to say, that the 20th century has been the bloodiest one in history thus far.

MEDICINE:
A MANIFESTATION OF THE
PSYCHOLOGICAL IMMUNE SYSTEM

While fire, tools, weapons, and shelter are outgrowths of our genetically programmed attempt to survive, we must also look at the practice of medicine as another manifestation of our push to survive, sometimes referred to as our will to live. As Norman Cousins states in his book Anatomy of an Illness, "the life-force may be the least understood force on earth." Cousins was given a one-in-five hundred chance of recovering from the condition called anykylosing spondylitis, a disorder in which the connective tissue in the spine progressively disintegrates which is considered incurable. But Cousins did not accept this prognosis, He used, and wrote about using humor as a healing tool. Based on his experience, he envisions that "medical researchers may discover that the human brain has a natural drive to sustain the life process and to potentiate the entire body in the fight against pain and disease."[32]

Although the earliest medical records go back some 4,000 years to a Sumerian clay tablet,[33] our ancestors, most probably, tried to help each other with injuries and illnesses long before that. Some evidence exists that Neandertals cared for members with fractured bones until they got better and could resume their normal activities.[34]

Helping members within a family, clan, or tribe makes good evolutionary sense, especially when it comes to mothers caring for injured or sick children. Although our hominid ancestors are all extinct, many of them were very successful in terms of survival time. Homo habilis survived for at least a half-million years;

Homo erectus for more than a million years; and the Neandertals for at least 100,000 years. Homo sapiens have been around for an estimated 130 thousand years.[35] Our urge to protect, preserve, and enhance our lives and physical well-being is still driving us to develop more effective medical interventions to prolong our lives and those of people we love and hold dear.

Early records show that physicians washed wounds, made poultices, and used bandages. Wounds were bathed in beer and hot water; poultices were made from materials such as pounded pine, prunes, wine dregs, and lizard dung. In fact, a list of 230 such concoctions was found in the remains of an Assyrian pharmacy.[36] One prehistoric medical practice involved cutting a small hole in the skull to treat headaches, epilepsy, and some forms of mental illness. Medical procedures were used together with incantations, sorcery, and appeals to the gods. The Ancient Egyptians, for example, performed surgical procedures on the outside of the body and also used sorcerers and exorcists to fight the evil of the disease. The ancient Hebrews believed disease resulted from displeasing God, but the Hebrews also excelled in the area of public health. Ancient Chinese medicine used acupuncture, and Chinese physicians attempted to cure diseases by restoring harmony and balance between the two opposing yet complementary forces of yin and yang.[37] They still do.

In times of famine, earthquake, or pestilence, ancient people turned to religion. Under the Byzantine emperors, for example, priests and doctors were one and the same. Disease was seen as a punishment resulting from sin or a lapse from the purity of religious life.[38] Our need to survive runs deep, and fear can take us on paths that make us seem irrational and barbaric. The Black Death, for instance, which ran rampant in Europe around 1300 A.D., was a type of bubonic plague caused by the microbe Pasteurello pestis , which lived in fleas that inhabited the black rat. When the fleas bit a person, the microbe was passed on. This particular plague was probably the greatest European catastrophe in history. Historians believe that some 24 million people died, which, at that time, comprised about a quarter of the European population. To many, the disease seemed to be supernatural in origin-a punishment from a higher power upon unknown sinners for unknown crimes. So, culprits were sought. First nobles came under suspicion, then cripples, and then Jews. The Jews were suspected of purposely spreading plague by contaminating wells and putting imagined poison in houses and on persons. As a result, reprisals started at Chillon on Lake Geneva in 1348 and spread to Basel, Bern, Freiburg, and Strassburg. At Basel and Freiburg all known Jews were herded into large wooden buildings and burned to death. At Strassburg, over two thousand were reported to have been hanged on a scaffold set up in the Jewish burial ground. The carnage was halted only after Pope Clement VI issued two bulls declaring the Jews innocent. The world had to wait until 1884 before the causative pathogen, Pasteurello pestis, was discovered.[39]

It wasn't until the Seventeenth century that the existence of germs was revealed by the microscope. This led to greater emphasis on cleanliness, and over the centuries sanitation, hygiene, and public health have played a greater and greater role in keeping disease under control. However, even in the Twentieth century, where crowded and unsanitary conditions prevailed, outbreaks of diseases could be devastating. Surat, in India, for example, experienced an outbreak of pneumonic plague in September 1994. Within six weeks the Indian government had over 6,000 suspected cases on its hands. At least fifty six deaths occurred, and 400 cases were confirmed by lab tests. When people in Surat heard the news, nearly half a million residents fled the city. This type of outbreak could occur in a city like Surat because half of its two million people live in squalid shantytowns with no sewers and no running water, making the city perfect breeding ground for a microbial killer.[40]

Spurred on by our urge to survive, over centuries we humans have developed, programs and controls that have reduced the threats to our health and safety. In many countries there are drinking water standards, plumbing codes, exhaust emission controls, meat inspections for bacteria contamination, agencies to test drugs before they are marketed, vaccination programs to head off a multitude of diseases, medical schools to train physicians and licensing exams to ensure they are competent to practice on the public. Federal and state hospital regulations are further controls, and codes exist for food handling and preparation. When you think about it, our need for survival manifests itself in ways almost too numerous to list. It is with us every minute of every day, whether we're aware of it or not.

HEADING INTO THE FUTURE

We still have industrial, chemical and radioactive contamination to deal with. We still have violence against our persons from criminal acts, intentional and unintentional shootings, domestic violence, and accidents. We still have cancer, AIDS, Alzheimer's disease, and birth defects to work on. Recently a new epidemic of a disease called severe acute respiratory syndrome, or SARS, has emerged, which is being watched closely by the medical community so that the disease doesn't spread worldwide. We have a whole host of mental illnesses to contend with, many of which lead to striking out at others, and some that result in self-destructive acts such as self-mutilation and suicide. Some say the future looks bright; others say the future looks dim.

One of the bright spots seems to be the Human Genome Project whose goal was to decipher the human genetic blueprint by locating the 30,000 or so genes in our twenty three pairs of chromosomes and determining what proteins they control and what problems develop when they are altered or missing.[41] The sequencing of the human genome was completed in April 2003 and scientists are still working on identifying all the genes and their functions.[42] To help in the diagnosis of malformations and disease we have a multitude of imaging techniques such as ultrasound scanning, computerized axial topography (CAT), magnetic resonance imaging (MRI), and digital X-rays. Organ transplants have become fairly routine, and brain functioning is being studied more intensely with the development of brain electrical activity mapping (BEAM). While new drugs and new technologies are quieting some of our survival anxiety, people are also turning in large numbers to alternative medicine, meditation, and prayer. It seems that more than just survival of the body is at stake.

It is important to recognize that we are driven by long-standing evolutionary forces, foremost among them being the urge for survival. We have engaged our symbolic, conceptual, and creative abilities for our protection, preservation and enhancement. When different groups of people see each other as enemies or threats, like the immune system treats foreign antigens, each group uses its survival skills to neutralize the other. Unfortunately, our technological know-how is such that it takes ten minutes to train a ten-year-old to pull a trigger or detonate a bomb, whereas it takes ten years to train an adult to repair the injuries created by the bullets or bomb. Therefore, no matter how hard we try we cannot train as many healers as destroyers.

We are learning to better understand and control our biological immune system, but we still haven't recognized that we also have a psychological immune system that needs to be respected and understood.

CHAPTER II

Our Sense Of Self and Identity
Keeping Score and Protective Actions

BLAMING OURSELVES

"You've got to die," Anna wrote to herself. "You can't go on any longer. It's impossible! It's not worth going on any longer. Break some glass and cut your throat, that will do it once and for all."

With these words Anna tried to convey the turmoil that was going on inside of her, the turmoil that had put her into psychiatric hospitals several times already. She called herself names and evaluated herself in the most derisive manner possible. She called herself "dirty," "rotten," and "selfish."

In her letters to herself she continued the diatribe against herself as if she deserved it all and then some. She referred to herself as "dirty and sinful," as well as "oversexed." She used the

27

latter term in self-judgment because she felt her desires were much stronger than they should be. She condemned herself for not being satisfied with what she had and for the urge of wanting more.

Anna traced the accusing finger of her conscience back to her mother, who attempted to raise her in accord with Catholic Church doctrines. Her extramarital affair with John and her continued fantasies about him were proof to her that she was a perverted person. Yet she recalled that during the affair she had felt more desirable than she had ever felt before, and that John had never criticized or rejected or made her feel incompetent. She could not say the same for her husband. So her fantasies about John continued and so did her guilt and her evaluation of herself as perverted. Through the numerous cuts on her arms and her suicide attempts, Anna played out the dilemma of her feelings and her self-condemnation

And to make matters worse, she went out of her way to let other people including her doctors, know that she didn't need them or their assistance. One could not help but come to the conclusion that the reason she tried to show she didn't care was that she cared too much about what other people thought of her. It's one thing to condemn yourself, but it's another thing when someone else condemns you and reinforces your own self-condemnation.

Like all human beings, Anna developed her own ways of protecting her self-worth, even while she vilified herself and tore down her sense of worth. While it may seem strange that a "rational" being should be so full of contradictions and inconsistencies, that is exactly what appears to be the case.

What did Anna have to say about her husband, Brian, to whom she had been married for five years? She wrote to herself that she didn't deserve Brian; that he deserved more than she could give him. In fact, she believed that he didn't really love her because she was too dirty and awful, even though he said he did. She was not convinced that he meant what he said; and deep down inside, she thought, he really didn't mean it.

Anna asked herself how her husband could trust her again after all of the "awful things" she had done. Anna guessed that Brian was convinced that since she had cheated on him once, she would do it again. In actuality, she didn't trust herself and felt that if given the chance, she would do it again because the yearning for John was still very strong. She missed him and fantasized about him often. She still needed and wanted him very much. Unable to resist the temptation, she was convinced that she had made "a mess" out of her life, and that she would be better off "ending it all" so that she wouldn't have to deal with her shame and guilt, which she verbalized as "hurt" she "couldn't stand much longer." That's why she continually entertained the idea of "ending it all."

Anna felt ashamed of herself for having strong sexual feelings and guilty of playing out her feelings with John, thus becoming a woman who was cheating on her husband and violating the teachings of her church. She found it hard to get to sleep because she anticipated the nightmares she often had, like jumping off a tall building or lying on a railroad track with a train bearing down on her. As she put it, "It's awful to have dreams like that."

Through Anna's writings one could sense the struggle she had had trying to decide who she really was. It showed in the struggle between her conscience and her desire to feel fulfilled as a woman. Marriage was on the side of her conscience and her sexual needs were on the side of fulfillment. But Anna's struggle was not unique. It happens to a lot of women in our culture. If one's husband is seen as too critical, too demanding, or too controlling, then the desire to find someone else arises.

One fantasy of such women is that of a Prince Charming who is non-critical, non-rejecting and makes one feel competent and desirable. Indeed, doesn't everyone look for someone who will enhance his or her sense of worth, self-respect and sense of accomplishment? Generally this looks like what is going on, but individually and specifically people often make poor choices in their mates, and some pay with physical injury or their lives. Like Anna, it seems that most people are not one whole integrated person who is proud of him or herself all the time. Conscience and desire are not always on the same wavelength. The same could be said of conscience and ambition or moral values and greed. If we bring more than one person into the equation and talk about the desires, ambitions, and values of different families and different groups, we find even more divisive battle between the values of different groups. The competition between such groups can become quite heated and prolonged.

What happened inside Anna was not totally unique to her. She struggles, we all struggle! Luckily the battle doesn't always involve self-mutilation and attempted suicide. While these are not extremely rare, most of us don't take this particular route in expressing the battles with ourselves.

Some of us run away from ourselves through drugs or alcohol; some develop chronic anxiety or depression, and some become workaholics. I say "us" because I see all of us as one species occupying one planet, and all of us living on borrowed time. We differ from each other, it's true and we don't all share common beliefs, values, or culture. But we all judge ourselves and others as to worth, status, trustworthiness, and deserving or not deserving our respect.

If we don't like ourselves, it makes living more difficult. Jason, for example, like Anna, blamed himself for the way things turned out in his life. He had just lost the greatest love of his life and felt that if he had only been more of a man, Wendy, would not have broken up with him. In the year they had been together Jason had to pinch himself to make sure he wasn't dreaming and convince himself that Wendy wanted to be with him.

Jason said that he had never rated himself very highly, when compared to the athletes and popular boys in his high school. In fact, he said, as far back as he could remember he had suffered from an inferiority complex but tried to cover it up. He pretended to be "one of the guys" and tried not show his uneasiness around girls.

After he graduated he attended junior college and received training as a psychiatric technician. He was pretty proud of himself when he obtained his license. But even while attending college he saw girls who he was convinced would never be interested in him because he lacked the qualities that attractive men had. He had many fantasies of his dream girl, not the least of which was her good looks and her appeal to other men. He finally found his dream girl in Wendy, who was also training to be a "psych tech." Needless to say, he was devastated when she broke up with him, and this reinforced his self-image as not man enough to find and keep a really attractive woman.

Anna and Jason were two individuals who judged themselves in a very negative way-Anna, because she did something she wasn't supposed to do, and Jason because he lacked something he believed others had. Their stories bring home the fact that we never stop judging and evaluating ourselves. It goes on continuously like breathing, eating, and other processes of our bodies. Our sense of who we are is crucial to us and is never far from our awareness. Children's sense of self starts at a very young age, probably in the first year, with the touch and response of their parents. Then, with the recognition of their name and their sensitivity to parental treatment and statements such as "no," "don't do that," "good boy or good girl," " isn't she cute," etc., children begin to develop an internal picture of themselves. They soon take on the same evaluation of themselves that they have received from their parents. This process continues as the children meet other family members, who also send out messages of love, anger, competition, acceptance and rejection. The same process goes on when they meet non-family members and other children. It doesn't stop until their brains stop, because we have to have a sense of ourselves in order to be human. We may not approve of ourselves, and may wish that our views of ourselves would disappear. But they stay with us like our bodies. They are our identity!

BLAMING OTHERS

Part of establishing one's identity is comparing one's self to others. While we pass this process on to our children, they do it naturally by themselves. Their evaluations, however, don't have the color of our prejudices. They learn that from us and older peers. While negative self-evaluations influence how we act and can have devastating consequences, positive evaluations also influence our actions and can also determine the outcome of our lives. This is especially true if we feel we are being treated unfairly or that we are being blocked in our efforts to enhance our productivity, our livelihood, or our lives. Then our negative evaluations and our anger are directed at the perceived source of our mistreatment rather than at ourselves as in the cases of Anna and Jason.

Henry, as an example, worked for the post office and complained bitterly about how unfairly his supervisor treated him and the other postal workers. He informed me that he had complained to the postal workers' union, but his complaints had produced no results.

He felt that his supervisor was belittling him in front of other employees and assigning him punishing jobs. He maintained that he had spoken to a number of other employees who felt the same way about this supervisor, but when the moment of truth arrived to speak to higher authorities about the problem, the employees became frozen in speech and action. Henry began to develop strong fantasies of doing bodily harm to the supervisor and talked about what would happen if he got carried away. He concluded that he had too much to lose by carrying out his urges but they came close to becoming his obsession for he felt that his whole sense of worth and dignity was on the line. He believed he deserved better!

This same theme of deserving to be treated better was voiced in a speech by Albert Einstein in 1954.[1] He said,

> The existence and validity of human rights are not written in the stars....Those ideals and convictions which resulted from historical experience, from the craving for beauty and harmony, have been readily accepted in theory by man-and at all times, have been trampled upon by the same people under the pressures of their animal instincts. A large part of history is therefore replete with the struggle for these human rights, an eternal struggle in which a final victory can never be won. But to tire in that struggle would mean the ruin of society.

SELF-JUDGMENT AND PUNISHMENT

So while Anna perceived herself as a disgusting human being-but didn't want to hear this from anybody else-Jason saw himself as a poor excuse for a man. Henry believed that he deserved to be respected more and treated better by his supervisor-the kind of treatment Einstein felt belongs to all men. While they do not all see eye to eye with each other, they are all doing what every human being does no matter what his or her condition. All four are evaluating or judging themselves and others. While Anna and Jason seem to feel they deserve to judge themselves negatively, Henry believes that he deserves better. Einstein believes all men deserve better.

Since individuals judge themselves and others, it must follow that groups do the same thing because groups are composed of a lot of individuals who share some common characteristic, common experience or common purpose. The Penitentes of New Mexico, for example, are a group of religious zealots who continue to practice the rituals, now in a subdued form, of exorcising sin through physically induced suffering such as flagellation.[2] In bygone days, the sect used whips and other devices of torture to discipline themselves until physical suffering, bleeding, and sometimes death occurred. They believed that there is no salvation without suffering and that since most sins are inspired by the flesh they must be exorcised by way of the flesh. In principle, this type of self-mutilation is similar to what Anna did to herself when she cut up her arms. While she did not use cutting as a religious ritual, she did want to punish herself for her sins, and she appeared

35

to obtain some emotional relief by creating pain and suffering. Self-punishment on both the individual and group levels, while not always resulting in physical injury, is a pretty common form of discipline. It stems from the human process of self judgment-judgment of goodness and badness.

Judging ourselves as to how good or how bad we are or how well or badly we behave, are measures we use to evaluate our worth. This, in turn, determines what we feel we deserve and what we can expect from ourselves and others. The ups and downs of everyday life have the potential to produce both negative and positive evaluations of ourselves. We see our shortcomings and our strong points, our good traits and our bad traits, our rational and our irrational thoughts, our honest and dishonest statements and the pleasant or unpleasant manner in which we behave toward others. This is the running scorecard we keep, even if we are not always conscious of doing so. These evaluations are translated into feelings that reach our consciousness and color all of our perceptions. If you are asked about your demeanor or what is going on, you might answer, "Oh nothing, I'm just in a funky mood." And you may not be able to pick out a reason.

JUDGING OTHERS

The statements by Henry and Albert Einstein remind us that not only do we look at our own shortcomings and our own behavior, we also judge others as well. Most of us, in fact, keep a running tally of who did or didn't treat us fairly, who did or didn't show us respect, who did or didn't act selfishly in a relationship with us, and who did or didn't use or abuse us. The emotion of love has a way of becoming attached to people who we sense are treating us fairly, with respect, unselfishly, and who don't use or abuse us. In contrast, the feeling of hatred easily directs itself to people who we believe are treating us unfairly, with disrespect, who have acted selfishly in a relationship with us, or who have used or abused us.

I recall talking to a grieving mother who had just lost her nineteen year old son, Kevin, in a fight with another young man who was attending a junior college. It seemed that the college student had cut Kevin off while driving home from school. Kevin apparently let the student know, via hand gestures, that he was not too pleased by this. After several more hand gestures were exchanged between them, Kevin followed the other young man home, where they got out of their cars and confronted each other. The college student, feeling the need to protect himself at all costs, pulled out a knife and stabbed Kevin in the chest. Unfortunately, the knife found its mark and killed Kevin. His grieving mother acknowledged that her son had a "hot temper" and was quick to take offense, but her loss was not lessened by this reflection. She ended her conversation with me by asking, "When will kids learn that some things are not a matter of life and death?"

From his mother's standpoint, Kevin became offended at being cut off by the other young man and also became offended at the hand gestures sent back to him. One could say that Kevin took the actions of the college student personally. All of us have probably said, at some time in our life to another individual, "don't take it so personally." Or we may have said that a statement, gesture or action was not meant to be personal. But what if that which is said or done is sensed as an insult? How can someone avoid taking it personally?

The answer is, you can't help taking something personally if you perceive it as an insult. However, what we do about it afterwards depends on how intensely the psychological injury is felt, our own temperament, what is at stake for us, and many other personal considerations. Going back to my own childhood, I recall that who you looked at and the way you looked at them carried significance for your personal safety. I must have heard the confrontation,"Who you looking at?" or "What the hell are you staring at?" hundreds of times. Each time the question was asked it had a decidedly threatening tone, which I sensed rather quickly. If the individual was much bigger than me or looked too tough, I would look away or say something like, "Sorry, I wasn't staring at you." However, if I felt I could meet the challenge I would say, "I'm looking at you! So what?" I knew these were fighting words and would be taken as such.

DEFENDING STATUS AND REPUTATION

As can be seen by Kevin's tragedy, our perception of insults and how we react to them can have grave consequences. I recognized this as a kid when I was challenged by the question "Who I was looking at?" Most kids are attuned to the consequences of calling someone's bluff or challenging someone else's tough stance. Self-image, self-worth, and personal safety all get tied up with our actions. When I was young it was mostly males who challenged each other physically. Now it seems that females also get into fist fights and use physically aggressive means to handle insults and challenges which were once almost exclusively the domain of males.

Part of the changing values of females who have taken on this tough and aggressive stance seems related to the rise of gang activity and gang aggressiveness. Many gangs are composed of alliances among individuals of the same ethnic background within a given neighborhood. Its members have the task of proving to the rest of the gang how tough they really are-girls included!

Belonging to a gang can give members a feeling of pride, status, and reputation. However, acceptance of the gang's code of conduct usually includes defending the territory of the gang, defending the gang's reputation or "honor," engaging in risky or illegal activities, and avenging the injury or death of other gang members. The intensity of gang membership, the code of silence, and the willingness of members to take the law into their own hands often baffle authorities. But one must remember that the emotional attachments to reputation, pride and status go back a long way in human history.

Not too long ago there was a drive-by shooting at a high school that resulted in the injury of a student. Needless to say, school was disrupted, students met in groups to talk about what happened, and the police came on campus to investigate the incident. Emotions were running pretty high, and the principal called in counselors to help the students cope with their feelings. I was one of the counselors.

Many of the students stated that they knew the identity of the attackers but were reluctant to reveal their names to the police. They stated that the attackers were from a nearby city and did the drive-by shooting to enhance their reputation among several gangs in their city. Some of the friends of the victim, who were affiliated with a gang of their own, talked of taking revenge for the attack. They were incensed to think that the attackers believed the shooting would intimidate their local gang. The longer they talked, the more it became evident that a gang code was involved in handling such an incident. The code required the local gang to handle the incident itself without involving the police or other authority figures. "Don't worry, we'll handle it in our own way and within our own time," they told me and the other counselors.

Silence and revenge seem to permeate gang members' code of conduct. Members who break this code are looked down upon, ostracized, and become gang targets themselves. Thus the self-respect of gang members and their acceptance by other members are strong incentives to live by the code. Revenge and retribution seem to be accepted reactions to invasions of territory, insults to gang members, challenges from other gangs, and injury or death of gang members by other gangs. Because of strong ethnic affiliations in particular neighborhoods, children develop part of their identity from their street friends, who may be gang members.

To non-gang members and the public at large, a gang's code of conduct and the pride of its members may seem repulsive and indicative of immaturity, at the least, and training for future criminal behavior. Thus the police, backed up by the public, have taken a strong stand against the activities of gangs, including tagging. In addition, gangsta rap and the record companies that sponsor and support it have come under fire.

Roger Hernandez, a syndicated columnist, wrote an editorial about the social milieu surrounding gangsta rap. This is what he had to say:[3]

> Performers don't tell us about violence to move against it, but to proclaim it as an integral part of their cultural identity. And it's not only violence they embrace; gangsta rap is a celebration of vulgarity, illiteracy, and inarticulateness. Gangsta rappers are, in short, proud to be stupid.

Hernandez goes on to say that the culture of the street is the real hurdle children have to jump over and that rap music glamorizes street culture. He sees identity and self-image at the heart of the matter, believing that the values kids internalize and which make up their self-image determine their actions.

He goes on to write,

> Self-identity is at the root of the crises. Street culture boils down to pride about being a hoodlum. Kids who fall prey to this mentality do not see themselves as part of a larger society, but as renegades. They consider themselves heir

to nothing but the street tradition of looking and acting tough. They bristle with ethnic pride that only cloaks a deep sense of inferiority toward the rest of the world.

So, gang X with its tough territorial, ethnic identity, says to gang Y, "Who do you think you are, acting toward us in the way you are? We have pride; we won't let you get away with this. We have a right to retaliate and get revenge." In turn, gang Y says the same thing to gang X. Then society, with its legal codes and parental identity, says to the gangs, "You can't act that way within our territory; you can't take the law into your own hands and hurt innocent victims. Who do you think you are, acting that way? We have a right to retaliate against you, take our own revenge and punish you. Maybe that will teach you a lesson about who's in charge and who has more power."

How Social Standards Affect Self Judgments

While society believes that gangs deserve to be judged harshly and condemned for their behavior, it has favorable judgments about other organizations and individuals. The community takes pride, for example, in local sport teams or individual athletes who go on to play in state tournaments, and even more pride if they win titles.

Sports competition between schools in the nearby cities, counties, and states is readily supported by society because the participants all compete according to the same adult-supervised rules. Winning is the goal, and team members feel elated when they win and dejected when they lose. Pride, honor and self-esteem are involved in these games, not only for the participants but also for the schools and communities they represent. The same pride is also involved in non-athletic tournaments, as is the emotional intensity of trying to win.

An article in the local newspaper,[4] for instance, told about the California Academic Decathlon, in which forty two teams from different high schools competed with each other. Although a local team didn't win, the paper reported the emotional reaction of a local high school placing higher than they had anticipated. This is how the paper reported the event,

> At Saturday's award ceremony following two days of rigid academic testing, the nine … High School[5] students and their two coaches stared nervously at one another as the names of the top 10 finishers were announced. As the sixth-place winner was read, the … High School team hung their heads dejectedly, looking at one another with consolation, confident they wouldn't place higher than eighth or ninth place. But in the split second following their fifth-place announcement, heads shot up, eyes opened in shock and seats slid back as the celebrating students leapt to their feet, embracing one another. "I just can't believe it," said the team coach[6]. "I thought

we'd place in the top 10, but when they announced 10th
through 6th I thought it was all over."

To the coach, the victory was even sweeter given the high
level of competition for the event. "Fifth place is extraordinary,"
the coach said. One of the team members summed up his feeling
thusly, "It's an incredible ego boost to know things about the world
you never knew before. The reward isn't the competition, but the
knowledge you walk away with." According to the paper, this
included testing in mathematics, science, language and literature,
fine arts, and social science, as well as in essay writing, speech,
and interview skills. Quite a contest!

As in this newspaper article, we are bombarded daily with people, events, and stories that rise to the status of newsworthiness and
reflect social judgments about what is acceptable, unacceptable, remarkable, noble, or disgusting. This bombardment is certainly one
avenue by which we become familiar with the standards we use to
judge ourselves and others.

In another newspaper article, under the headline, "Police
laud man as 'hero'" the actions of a man who saved another
man's life are described.[7] It relates that Mr. H was traveling
with his fiancee just a week before his wedding when he saw
a man being stabbed by a woman on the side of the freeway.
He stopped his car, got out, and restrained the knife-wielding
woman. The man he saved had already been stabbed more
than twenty times before he intervened. A police sergeant
who evaluated the event commented, "He's a true citizen hero.

Certainly, he put himself in immediate danger. She could have turned the knife on him." The sergeant probably speaks for a lot of people who would agree that Mr. H. deserves to be called a hero.

If children hear about the above story, they know what someone called a "hero" does. Saving another person's life is then recorded on their ongoing scorecard as an act of heroism. Some of the standards children are exposed to become internalized, and children then apply these standards to their own actions-just as the member of a gang does ; just as the member of a football team does; just as the member of a debating team or a member of the faculty does. We evaluate ourselves and others by way of these standards. Sometimes we are repulsed by someone else's behavior and feel that they deserve all the dishonor and punishment we can give them. This is the case for the bomber of the Oklahoma City federal building. Other times we are impressed with the behavior of someone else and feel that they deserve all the honor and gratitude we can bestow on them. A case in point might be the parents of Nicholas Green.

As the story unfolds, the Green family, consisting of the father, the mother and seven year old Nicholas, were driving to Sicily during a vacation in Italy. From what is known, along the way their car was fired upon by highway bandits. The parents managed to escape uninjured, but a bullet struck Nicholas in the head as he slept on the back seat. Nicholas was taken to a nearby hospital, where he died. The parents, after learning of their son's death, donated his organs to people in Italy in need of them. Nicholas's organs were transplanted to five different people. When one of the most respected commentators in Italy, Enzo Biagi, heard of the tragedy and the actions of the parents, he wrote an open letter on the front page of the Milan daily *Corriere della Sera*.

The letter said:

> I must, I want, to thank you; Not only for the transplants, but for a lesson. Of generosity, of composure. With us, violence is an ancient evil and marks many destinies. This land, famous for history, beauty, art, suffers from an invincible cruelty, which hides behind the oleanders, the sycamores, among the ruins...and which at night strikes a little sleeping Nicholas.

The city to which the wounded Nicholas was taken made the Green family honorary citizens because of their altruism. Provincial officials established a $1,200 elementary school scholarship in Nicholas's honor. Rome honored the family with a gold medal, and an association of parents of children with heart disease made the Greens honorary members. The story also made headlines in the United States.[8]

THE INTERACTION BETWEEN NATIONS AND INDIVIDUALS

It can be seen from this story that the actions of individuals and groups can and do have an effect on a nation's reputation and conscience. But sometimes the actions of individuals and groups are taken as signs of disrespect to the authorities, which in turn may be seen as the first sign of a threat to those in power. This can produce a violent counter-reaction from authorities, who will not and cannot tolerate any sign of disrespect. This is poignantly brought out by anthropologist Jack Weatherford in his book *Savages and Civilization*. Writing about the rise of gangs, their tribalism, and their illegal activities, he gives his eyewitness account of the Chinese authorities' reaction to this phenomenon. He writes,

> One night in the Chinese city of Xian, I witnessed the extent to which Chinese authorities proved willing to go to limit crime in their cities. I saw a major public spectacle near the center of town as a noisy crowd gathered around a dozen young men with shaved heads. The young men stood with terrified eyes on the back of a truck before the crowd. Signs on the side of the truck proclaimed their various crimes which they had to confess in public. At the end of the ceremony of public confession and shame, the police drove the young men to the edge of town and shot them, each one with a single bullet to the back of the head. The family of each executed criminal then had to pay a token fine of a few cents to pay for the bullet.

What can you say to absolute authority that holds your life and death in its hands? Can you say, "Look, I may have broken some of your rules, but don't take it personally. It was never meant to be personal, and you still have ruling status in my mind. I am still mindful of your power, stature, and leadership. My actions were not meant to challenge your authority."

As previously noted, if your actions are seen as an insult and challenge to someone- authority figures included-then your actions are going to be taken personally. "How dare you act like that toward me (or the country I rule). Who do you think you are?" is the response you are likely to receive. Rulers have a way of making laws against actions that threaten their power or insult their authority. In many countries, this assures that leaders go unchallenged in rigged elections in which opposition parties are banned.

Paul Weiss, a former Sterling Professor of Philosophy at Yale University, coined the word "idiocide," which literally means killing someone's sense of self or worth. He maintains that this happens too often in our societies, as individuals are deprived of either their stature or their status.[10] Loss of stature occurs when events such as starvation, torture or murder affect people individually. Loss of status takes place when individuals are deprived of their opportunity to carry out their roles in society.

In Dr. Weiss' own words,

> Indeed, every means of human destruction from genocide to war, no matter what the occasion, excuse,

explanation, or benefit, is inevitably idiocidal, reducing
the stature of an individual, making him less than a
human can be and should be. There is a denial of status
when an individual is brought down or kept from the
position he normally or rightfully occupies, turning
him into a victim, a hostage, a prisoner, a neglected or
alienated member of society, cut off from the opportunity
to survive, to maintain a level already achieved, or even
to grow-thereby making his promise meaningless.

Since one's sense of self and sense of worth are part and parcel
of one's identity, idiocide is really the killing of one's identity. Not an
insignificant event! Dr. Weiss believes that society has an obligation
to prevent acts of idiocide, reduce the effects of these acts when
they do occur and help people recover their status or compensate
them for its loss. He does not, however, differentiate between
society's obligation to its members who are in good standing and
its obligation to its members who do not follow its rules and laws.
Fairly recently, for example, the Supreme Court of the United States
ruled in the case of Bennis vs. Michigan[11] that private property
(in this case a car) in which or upon which illegal activity occurs
can be seized by the police and confiscated...even if the owner of
the property was unaware that illegal activity was taking place.

Using Dr. Weiss's concepts, does not this law lower the status of
the property owner who didn't know illegal activity was occurring
in or on his property? Isn't he or she being treated in the same way

as a property owner who knows illegal activities are occurring? Is this not a judgment of who deserves and who doesn't deserve to keep his property? Indeed, aren't all social norms and laws ways of judging who deserves to be treated with respect and who deserves to be punished?

Making judgments about ourselves and others and acting on those judgments seems to be the nature of us human beings and the societies we create. Our status and stature depend on those judgments, but also affect them. For example, if we judge ourselves as incompetent and others do the same, this reinforces our own sense of self. However, if we judge ourselves as competent and others judge us as incompetent, we would question the other judgment more.

When we consider Einstein's assertion that human beings have certain rights that should be respected by society and Weiss' assertion that society has an obligation to prevent acts that demean its members, we end up with the conclusion that the way individuals attain and maintain their status and stature is by having the freedom and means to accomplish their goals and aspirations.

Too often, however, members of a society are divided into classes and a different status is assigned to each class, with the higher-ranking classes getting more privileges and the lower-ranking classes being exploited more. A child who grows up in this type of system has a tendency to adopt a self-image and a sense of worth based on his rank, because other people tend to treat him as if his worth were his rank.

Since children are the most vulnerable members of society, they can most easily be taken advantage of unless protected by adults and unless this protection is sanctioned by society. A 1995 Amnesty International report, for instance, stated that there are more than 7.5 million children in Pakistan who are held as bonded laborers, despite government legislation passed in 1992 to outlaw that practice.[12]

Iqbal Masih was one of these children. He was apparently sold as a slave to carpet manufacturers in order to work off a family debt. This happened when he was four years old! Carpet makers like children because their tiny fingers are able to do the intricate work demanded in making carpets. So, like millions of other children, Iqbal was forced to work twelve hours a day to pay off his family's debt.

When Iqbal was ten years old, a representative of the Bonded Labor Liberation Front (BLLF) organization-established to end indentured servitude-came to his town. Iqbal asked some questions and found out that he had some rights as a citizen of Pakistan.

After learning this, Iqbal refused to go back to work and obtained a letter from a lawyer who worked for the BLLF specifying his right not to be in bondage. The letter was given to the carpet maker for whom he worked. Iqbal then enrolled in a special school set up by the BLLF for children freed from bondage. He participated in marches in support of children's rights and spoke to groups about his ordeal at home and abroad.

In December of 1994, Iqbal was named the recipient of the Youth in Action Human Rights Award sponsored by the Reebok

Foundation. He was presented with a $15,000 scholarship and went to Boston, Massachusetts, to accept the award. During his acceptance speech he stated that he planned to use the scholarship to get a law degree. The next day Iqbal went to visit the Broad Meadows Middle School in Quincy, just outside Boston. There, at a school assembly, he had the opportunity to tell his story to American children his own age. The students got a chance to talk to him after the assembly and found him to be a likable and fascinating member of their own age group.

After his visit to Broad Meadows Middle School, Iqbal went back to his home in Pakistan. On April 16, 1995, Easter Sunday, he was killed by an assassin's bullet as he rode his bicycle outside his grandmother's home. So, at age twelve, Iqbal Masih became one of the youngest victims of indentured servitude in Pakistan. The Amnesty International report stated, "It is widely believed that the child was killed because, though barely an adolescent, he had already become one of Pakistan's most outspoken and articulate human rights activists."

Iqbal's death had a profound effect on the students of Broad Meadows. They decided to build a Pakistani school in his honor. They enlisted the aid of a T-shirt printing company, Amnesty International, and Senator Edward Kennedy, and they created an Iqbal Masih home page on the World Wide Web. As of the summer of 1995, they had raised over $2,000. Thus, while Iqbal was initially treated as child with no rights and no status and later as a threat to the industry of indentured servitude, he was treated with great honor by the Reebok Foundation and the students of Broad Meadows Middle School. Most people would also agree that Iqbal raised his own stature by standing up for his own and other children's rights, for which he gave his life.

It seems we really can't get away from continually judging ourselves and others and then acting on our judgments. It appears that these judgments are based on who we are, and who we are depends on these judgments. Henry, for instance, believed his supervisor treated him unfairly and felt he deserved more respect; the friends of the student injured in the drive-by shooting felt their status and honor were being challenged and believed revenge was justified; the students in the Academic Decathlon felt proud of their accomplishments, as did their coach, and the community paper made them newsworthy; Mr. H. was honored for saving the life of another man; the parents of Nicholas Green were praised and esteemed for donating the organs of their murdered son; the Chinese authorities felt justified in killing a dozen young men for breaking their laws, which in effect showed disrespect for the rules of the authorities; and someone or some group felt justified in killing Iqbal for speaking out too boldly for children's rights. In effect, the judgment process appears to be the mechanism by which we regulate our sense of self and our self-worth, both of which help make up our identity. Sometimes even our lives are sacrificed for our identity.

A REASON TO KILL

Arthur Koestler, a novelist and writer on scientific topics, has an interesting take on why we kill each other.[13] He proclaims:

Within a given species, conflicts are settled by ritualized forms of combat which, owing to some powerful inhibitory mechanism, nearly always stops short of inflicting lethal injuries. A hawk killing a field-mouse can hardly be accused of homicide. In man, however, the biological taboo against the killing of conspecifics (our own species) is singularly ineffective. But if we agree that something might have gone wrong in the evolution of our species, and search for an explanation, we always get the dusty answer that all evil stems from the selfish, aggressive tendencies in human nature.

This is the explanation that has been offered by Hebrew prophets, Indian mystics, Christian moralists, by contemporary psychologists and in popular tracts like Lorenz's *On Aggression*. But speaking in all humility, I find this answer unconvincing and without support in the historical record. What the record indicates is that the part played by violence for selfish personal motives has always been negligibly small compared with the numbers massacred in unselfish devotion to one's tribe, nation, church or leader, in the name of metaphysical or abstract causes.

Koestler's notion of devotion can easily be translated into the bonds that bind humans to each other in groups and from which our sense of self, self-worth and identity flow. He believes this explains why soldiers kill. He states,

> Soldiers do not hate. They are frightened, bored, sex starved, homesick. They fight the mostly invisible, impersonal enemy either because they have no choice, or out of loyalty to King and Country, to the true religion the righteous cause. They are motivated not by aggression, but by devotion.

While Koestler has some good arguments for his belief that loyalty rather than aggression accounts for people killing people, he doesn't seem to consider what happens when the king, country, or group to which one feels devotion comes under attack. Then anger, rage, and murder can and do result from our outrage at someone daring to threaten or destroy our beloved country or group. It is like someone trying to destroy our family or our home.

A case in point might be the not-too-distant massacres in Rwanda of Tutsis by Hutus. The events appeared to be triggered by the shooting down of the plane in which the presidents of Rwanda and Burundi were flying. Radio broadcasts sponsored by Hutu political organizations blamed Tutsis for the assassinations although the assailants were really unknown.[14] A bloodbath followed. A grizzly account of the murder of some Tutsi children was printed in the newspaper.[15] The newspaper reported that peasants from around Kigali, who were rounded up by the Rwandan Patriotic Front, gave detailed accounts of the "horrors" they helped carry out in their village.

For instance, Juliana Mukankwaya, the mother of six children, stated that she and other Hutu women rounded up the children of fellow villagers they regarded as enemies. Then, with gruesome resolve, they bludgeoned the stunned youngsters to death with large sticks. The paper quoted her as saying, "They didn't cry because they knew us." The slightly built thirty five-year-old woman maintained that she and the other Hutu women were doing the murdered children a favor, since they were orphans who faced a hard life. She stated, "Their fathers had been butchered with machetes and their mothers had been taken away to be raped and killed."

The murder of these children could be seen as acts of Hutu women loyal to the Hutu tribe carrying out the wishes of their leaders. They could also be seen as Hutu women carrying out revengeful acts because the president of Rwanda, who was a Hutu, had been assassinated and they believed the Tutsis were responsible. A third possible explanation is that the acts of the women were a combination of loyalty to the Hutus and revenge against the Tutsis. Arthur Koestler's point that humans kill out of devotion far more often than because of selfish and aggressive tendencies would be perfectly valid if the addendum were added that devotion can also lead to murderous rage if those to whom we are devoted come under attack. If it is acknowledged that part of our human identity comes from the individuals and groups we love, care about, and are bonded with, it can be seen that an attack on these individuals or groups is considered as an attack on ourselves and treated as such.

In fact, at times an attack is treated as if it were an attack on something greater than ourselves. In that case we act as though to give one's life for the group or the group's cause is the greatest glory of all. The added incentive of going to paradise or heaven doesn't hurt. Our actions are believed to enhance our self-worth, self esteem, status and stature in the eyes of the group. We become martyrs and are convinced we bring honor to the group and further its cause, which is also our cause.

So it was during the medieval Crusades which lasted almost 200 years and saw thousands of martyrs die for a religious cause. History portrays the Children's Crusade of 1212 as the most heartbreaking event of the period.[16] Hundreds of European children, mostly from France and Germany, went forth with religious zeal to conquer the Mohammedan armies which held the Holy Land. Most, apparently, didn't even get close, but died of disease, starvation, or the hardships of the long march. Others were captured and sold as slaves.

So it was also in the Second World War when kamikaze pilots from Japan went on suicide missions in airplanes loaded with explosives, crashing into United States warships in the pacific. They died, so it was believed, for the glory of Japan and its emperor. They were heroes to the people of Japan because they sacrificed their lives and chose "death before dishonor," a phrase that resonated well with the history of Japan.

While visiting San Francisco in the 1980s, I was riding in a taxi and struck up a conversation with the driver, who identified himself as an Afghan. He said he had made numerous trips back and forth between the United States and Afghanistan. With the money he made in the United States, he helped the mujahedeen fight their war with the Soviet Union, which then occupied his country. He said emphatically that the Soviet Union could never win the war in his country because the mujahedeen were not afraid to die. He stated they all knew that if they died they would go to paradise. The name "mujahedeen," in fact, means "fighters of the faith," and they believed God was on their side. So, my driver asked rhetorically, how can you conquer a people who are not afraid to die? His firm belief in their cause came across loud and clear. He felt that his countrymen were at a higher level than the soldiers of the Soviet Union, who had no great cause on their side. Considering the fact that the Soviet Union eventually withdrew lends validity to his belief.

So it is with Hamas, a militant Islamic group that sends out suicide bombers to blow themselves up in buses and shopping centers crowded with Israeli civilians. Their immediate objective, we are told, is to derail the peace process between Israel and the Palestine Liberation Organization. Their final objective is to destroy Israel. While the members of Hamas have religious fervor, they also have a deep hatred of Israel based on some rather stereotyped and false beliefs that are promulgated by the organization. For example, in just days before he strapped himself with explosives and drove his bicycle into an Israel checkpoint, killing himself and three soldiers, a Hamas Suicide bomber told an interviewer, "They claim they are the chosen people of God. But, in fact, Israel wants to destroy the world. They want to destroy American society, French society, British society. They want to destroy the whole world. But we believe Israel will be destroyed by Moslems. That is what the Koran says. That is not just a theory. It is reality."[17]

When people have a cause they consider to be of life-and-death proportions, their whole identity is bound up with the cause and many are willing to give up their own lives to serve the cause. The cause may be the protection of their families, their land, their rights, or their self-respect. Such a group of people wrote the following:

> We, therefore, the representatives of the United States
> of America in General Congress assembled, appealing
> to the Supreme Judge of the world for the rectitude of
> our intentions, do, in the name, and by the authority
> of the good people of these colonies, solemnly publish
> and declare: That these United Colonies are, and of
> right ought to be, free and independent states; they are
> absolved from all allegiance to the British Crown, and

that all political connections between them and the state
of Great Britain is, and ought to be totally dissolved;
and that, as free and independent States, they have full
power to levy war, conclude peace, contract alliances,
establish commerce, and to do all other acts and things
which independent States may of right do. And for the
support of this declaration, with a firm reliance on the
protection of Divine Providence, we mutually pledge
to each other our lives, our fortunes, and our sacred
honor.

This, of course, is the last paragraph of the Declaration of
Independence, which was issued in 1776. It is of interest to note
what the founders considered of utmost importance in their pledge
to each other-their life, their property, and their sense of honor or
worth. While one can see and touch live people and their possessions,
"sacred honor" is a concept and, as such, cannot be seen and touched.
But it was just as important to the signers as life and possessions.

We protect our worth and identity (honor, pride, status, etc.)
with the same evolutionary zeal with which we protect our life,
our physical well-being, our property, and our possessions. Thus
an attack on one's identity is just as painful as an attack on one's
body or an attack on one's prized possessions. Attacks on any of
these can be, and oftentimes are, met with the same intensity of
self-defense and retaliation.

The built-in alertness to threats on life, physical well-being, property, possessions, sense of self and identity, and our emotional reactions to such threats, constitute the essence of the psychological immune system. This will be explored in more detail in later chapters.

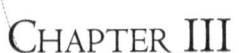

CHAPTER III
Evolutionary Considerations
Our Genes and Our Ancestors

LEADERS AND FOLLOWERS

Even though the Declaration of Independence declares, "We hold these truths to be self-evident: that all men are created equal," there were class distinctions in the various states at the time of its signing. Slaves were on the bottom rung, and moneyed gentry at the top rung. There are still class distinctions in the United States as well as in every other country in the world. This has been the state of affairs since at least the dawn of recorded history and, more than likely, before written language was conceived. Our perceptual ability to make distinctions among ourselves and our conceptual ability to classify everything certainly lay the groundwork for assigning certain people and groups to inferior positions and other people and groups to superior positions.

Our competitive nature and our tendency to follow those people who exert more authority and leadership are traits that tend to perpetuate class distinctions.

Many species of animals seem to exhibit patterns of dominance and submission in their groups, with the more dominate animals becoming the leaders. Scientists and naturalists, while they don't always agree with each other, have observed a hierarchy among many species. Robert Dantzer, a specialist in the scientific study of emotion, believes that this state of affairs is characteristic of species that compete for territory and limited resources.[1] This includes the primates-lemurs, apes, chimpanzees, and humans as well.

Dr. Robert Russell, who has extensively studied the nocturnal and diurnal lemurs of Madagascar, has reported some interesting observations in his book *The Lemur's Legacy* about the patterns of dominance, rank, and status in their family groups, known as troops. He maintains that the early primates of some thirty to fifty million years ago, of which modern Madagascar lemurs are descendants, displayed a social order of female dominance, stable matrilines, and seasonally aggressive, migratory males.[2]

The diurnal lemurs on Madagascar also display a social order of female dominance, with the most dominant called the alpha female and the most submissive called the omega female. The rest of the female troop, about a dozen or so, are ranked between these two extremes. The three or four closest in rank to the alpha female, the beta females, form a coalition with the alpha female. The coalition is the controlling force in the troop, which is made up of a couple of dozen lemurs (including males) and their offspring. The males have their own bachelor subgroup, which is also divided up from the most dominant to the most submissive; but the bachelor group is submissive to the female coalition throughout most of the year. However, during the annual mating period in April the male ranking within the bachelor group falls apart. It appears to be every male for himself in trying to get a piece of the action.

Russell in his book describes the male lemur's arousal and mating behavior as follows:

> The helter-skelter that marks the male mating frenzy is almost unimaginable. For the males, dominance ranks are quickly and summarily abandoned. Formerly, high-ranking males find that their alpha or beta status is challenged continuously. Former alliances dissolve in the quest for a desirable female. Male consorts must continually defend their bond. Males square off against each other night and day. Tails flutter defiantly toward one another in spontaneous, provocative scent fights. Screams, chases, flailing limbs, swipes of razor-sharp fingernails, and slashes of stiletto- sharp canine teeth tear at both the flesh and the social fabric of the lemur troop.

Russell believes that some male lemurs get so caught up in asserting and defending their rank that mating becomes a secondary consideration. It is as though nature overdid it with male sex hormones, and this undermined the original purpose of the hormones.

In contrast to the mating frenzy of male lemurs, which jolts their status position, the coalition of alpha and beta females stays in control. They determine where the troop goes, when it will travel from one feeding and resting area to another, and they are the leaders in defending the troop's foraging area. Along with this responsibility also come the benefits of high rank and status. They get the best food and the safest resting place in the tree; they get to be groomed by a following of lower-ranking females and males, and their infants get preferential treatment from birth. Their female infants will most likely ascend to the top ranks of the troop when they reach maturity. Their male infants will likewise rise to the top of the bachelor group. Unfortunately, the low-ranking females of the troop are continuously harassed by the higher ranking females and thus are under constant stress. Their offspring are observers of this behavior and, apparently, fare no better with their own peers. It is of interest to contemplate how infants in the same troop can have such different experiences of reality by merely being born to mothers of different rank.

Among the early apes called dryopithecines, who were descendants of a transitional line of African lemurs, ranking patterns were also present. Dryopithecines are believed to have been the immediate ancestors of modern orangutans, gorillas, chimpanzees, and ape-men. Unlike lemurs, however, the change in their female estrus cycle from yearly to monthly triggered a year-round flow of testosterone in males. This produced the aggressive, dominance-posturing, rank-defending behavior so aptly described in the lemur males. As a result, the males eventually took over control of the social group's of dryopithecines and their decendents.

CHANGE FROM FEMALE TO MALE LEADERSHIP

In Russell's view, this transition from female to male domination tested the survival of those species in which there was constant, unrelenting male aggression that disrupted the social fabric of the troop. The species that survived apparently adopted three different strategies to deal with unrelenting male aggression. Ape societies of solitary males and females evolved, like modern orangutans; ape societies with a harem social order evolved, like modern African gorillas; and ape societies with male power coalitions evolved, like chimpanzees.

Male power coalitions among chimpanzees resemble the female power coalitions among the diurnal lemurs described by Russell. It consists of the most dominant individual, known as the alpha, backed up by one or more individuals, called betas. This ruling class, as it were, maintains order in the community through power, intimidation, and cunning. As an evolutionary experiment, the power hierarchy seems relatively successful because it maintains order in the community, and thus, has survival value for the species. Dr. Jane Goodall, who studied chimpanzee communities in Gombe, Tanzania, for thirty years, recounts a story in her book *Through a Window*, in which an alpha male's brother and coalition partner, Faben, vanished and left his brother, Figan, to fend for himself. During Faben's absence, Figan was challenged by groups of other males and didn't fare too well. Thus, there was a period when no single alpha male was in charge of the community. During this period a sexually popular female, known as Pallas, came into estrus. The following account by Dr.Goodall underscores the importance of a dominant leader.[3]

> It was during this troubled period that the sexually popular female, Pallas, came into oestrus again after losing an infant. And, with no clear-cut alpha, this caused almost total chaos among the males. Figan no longer had the power to take sole possession of a hot number like Pallas-nor had any of his rivals. And so almost every time one of the big males climbed her tree (for probably in sheer self-defence she spent most of her time above the ground) pandemonium broke out among the others. Either the daring suitor himself was chased up a tree and attacked by one or more of the males or, if he made it to his goal, the sight of the sexual act triggered aggressive outbursts among the spectators. And then there would be a brief spell of bedlam as

males displayed with bristling hair and furious scowls, hurling rocks and occasionally seizing and pounding some luckless female or adolescent who got in the way. Sometimes they engaged in brief but furious battles between themselves. Pallas herself was rarely a victim but she must, nevertheless, have suffered through any number of almost unbearably tense moments.

This description of the bedlam among chimpanzee males is much like the description of the mating frenzy among the diurnal lemurs of Madagascar. Since survival of the chimpanzee group depends on an alpha male being dominant enough to keep male aggression under control, it follows that the emergence of an alpha male is an extremely important event and that the power struggle to reach that position is a fierce one. And in fact this is the case! First the males have to challenge and dominate all the females in the community. Then they have to challenge the top- ranking males in the community. This is no easy feat, and the males have to practice their displays of intimidation and ferocity before they can wield them successfully.

One individual chimpanzee, Mike, even made use of empty four-gallon tin cans, which he hit and kicked ahead of him as he charged his rivals. According to Goodall, this imaginative and novel behavior succeeded in intimidating all the males, including chimps much larger than himself. Normally, however, rocks and branches are used as part of the display, as in Goodall's description of a display by the alpa male Figan.

> He developed an impressive charging display. This display serves to make a chimpanzee look bigger and more dangerous than he may actually be-his hair stands on end; he leaps up to shake the vegetation; he drags huge branches noisily along the ground, then hurls them ahead of him; he picks up and throws rocks with such vigour that they fly unpredictably ahead, behind or to the side; he stamps and slaps loudly upon the ground or some tree trunk; his lips are tightly compressed, pulling his face into a ferocious scowl. And the wilder and more impressive his display, and the more carefully it is planned and executed, the better his chance of intimidating his rivals without recourse to actual physical combat-during which he himself, as well as his opponent, might be injured.

Figan became a master at displaying at the crack of dawn, when the other chimps were still sleeping in their tree nests. Here is Goodall's description,

> Back and forth, up and down-Figan leapt from branch to branch, shaking the vegetation, snapping great

branches and, for good measure, pounding, from time to time, on some unfortunate subordinate. The confusion and the noise were unbelievable.

If emotional intensity indicates how important something is to an animal, and it does seem like a good indicator, then gaining status is very important to male chimpanzees. Other situations producing intense emotions include mothers protecting their infants, scouting parties defending their territory and attacking trespassers, males coercing females to accompany them, offspring becoming separated from their mothers, offspring being weaned from their mothers and the death of either the offspring or the mother.

SEARCHING FOR STATUS

I recall a teenager telling me a story about an incident that made her re-evaluate her importance to her father. She explained that when she was fifteen years of age she was allowed to come and go as she liked. She stated that she would come home at all hours of the morning and even though her mother or father was up, neither would say anything to her. She thought they were pretty "cool" parents, and she loved the freedom she had. She of course hung around with older kids, and she would drink beer and other alcoholic beverages with them and smoke marijuana. One night she came home somewhat high and walked into the room where her father was tending to his coin collection. She inadvertently bumped into the glass case where the coin collection was kept, disrupting slightly the orderliness of the coins. As she described it, her father came unglued. He raved and ranted, despite her apologies, well into the night. As she went to bed that evening the realization came to her that her father's coin collection meant more to him then she did. After all, he never raved and ranted about her late hours, her drinking, or the people she hung around with. The emotional impact of this revelation left her in a daze. Without a sense of belonging she left her home and never returned.

Kids can gain status by hanging around with an older and more experienced group, while adults can gain status by associating with people of high rank and power. Chimpanzees, who split off from the human evolutionary line about seven million years ago, also gain status by proxy. Faben, for example, associated closely with the alpha male Figan and was thus able to share Figan's sexual possessions and food and was treated with deference by the other chimps in the community. The same thing happened when a chimp named Humphrey became a close ally of Figan. The expression "rank has its privileges" seems to apply equally well to human and chimpanzee societies.

Just as chimpanzees have their high-ranking alpha male and his partners, humans have their pharaohs, kings, nobles, emperors, sheiks, dictators, czars, chiefs, prime ministers, and presidents. And if you think chimpanzee displays are awesome, think about some of the displays, past and present, of our leaders. Instead of shaking branches and throwing rocks, humans competing for leadership have thrown armies against each other. They have hurled insults at each other, engaged in shaking rumors and money at the public, and have been as underhanded and devious as the human mind can make them. And they have been experts at rationalizing their behavior. If nothing else, it shows how much more creative we are than chimpanzees. But it also shows that chimpanzees developed social rank and vicious competition for leadership long before we did. Are we just copycats, or is the evolutionary programming similar in chimpanzees and human beings?

OUR EVOLUTIONARY PROGRAMMING

Evidence shows that chimpanzees are closer to the human species than any other species on earth. Studies of the DNA of humans and chimpanzees have found a difference of between one and two percent. While this doesn't seem to be very much, it is apparently enough to give us our distinct human characteristics. One of these characteristics is the ability to create symbols for anything we can sense, think about, or feel. Another is our ability to manipulate these symbols in systematic ways to create understandable linear patterns, internally consistent and logical systems, and stylized visual patterns. Words are such symbols; numbers are such symbols; drawings, pictures and sculptures are such symbols; musical notations are such symbols. Language, mathematics, graphic design, construction, and artistic expression are the systems in which or by which these symbols can be and are manipulated. Thus, humans can write instructions, make maps, draw faces, make building plans, sculpt a horse, build rocket ships and create symphonic compositions.

Through the use of our symbols and the systems in which they are managed, we are able to conceptualize the world around us and ourselves, as well. A chimpanzee seems to have a rudimentary ability to use hand signals as symbols, make tools, and recognize that the image in a mirror is of itself and not that of another chimp. We, however, not only realize that the figure in the mirror is our self and not some other individual, but we go on to make judgments about our self, just as Anna did, and we may then feel guilty, ashamed, proud, or even awed by our self.

Thus a leader or ruler may regard himself or herself as someone above and beyond an alpha member of his group. For example, in the twenty-fourth century B.C. the Akkadian ruler Naramsin, the grandson of Sargon I, who subjugated Sumer and founded the first known empire, proclaimed himself to be lord of the world and put the cuneiform sign of divinity before his name.[4] The pharaohs of Egypt were also considered gods and all-powerful. Nor have they been the last rulers whose sense of power has dominated their sense of self.

REVENGE AND WAR

While chimpanzees do not make judgments about themselves in the same way humans do, they do seem to have a sense of fairness and a sense of loyalty, both of which can lead to retribution and revenge. Their actions have even been interpreted as warlike. Examples of these traits and behaviors have been noted by Dr. De Waal, who studied the world's largest chimpanzee colony, which is housed in the Arnhem Zoo in the Netherlands.[5] Retribution and revenge were also observed by Goodall.

De Waal uses the term "moralistic aggression" to describe aggressive behavior by a chimpanzee against other chimps who take more than they give, e.g. food, or who do not reciprocate in kind the type of support they have been given. As an example he sites a case in which a female supported male A against male B. Shortly thereafter, male B threatened this same female. She held out her hand to male A to help her against male B, but male A did not come to her defense. De Waal describes the reaction of the female: "Immediately, the female turned on male A, barking furiously, chasing him across the enclosure."

He also found that individuals who shared their food were less likely to encounter resistance when they requested food from others. This correlation between giving and receiving food seemed to hold regardless of the individual's position in the dominance order, thus making the behavior an embedded trait. De Waal also noted retribution by a chimp, against particular individuals who had previously acted out against him. It was as though the chimp, were "getting even."

After recording every instance, over a ten-year period, of an individual chimp intervening in a fight between two others, De Waal found that the chimp who was intervened against would reciprocate against the intervener when the chance arose. So, for instance, if A supported B against C, it was characteristic for C to support another chimp against A. It almost fits the expression so often heard among people, "what goes around, comes around." De Waal sums things up as follows:

> The reciprocity of harmful intervention behavior in chimpanzees indicates the existence of a so-called revenge system; that is, victims of a contra intervention by another individual tend to pay this individual back in kind. Although the calculated nature of these processes cannot be proven without experimentation, the phenomenon is in line with the emerging picture of chimpanzees as creatures capable of keeping mental records of social events and adjusting their behavior according to rules of reciprocity that apply to both beneficial and harmful acts.

Goodall recounts a series of events in the Gombe community that appears to fit with De Waal's findings. In 1974 the community, which included fourteen adult males, began to divide. One group of six males moved farther south, leaving eight adult males in the original group. Two years after the first signs of the split, the chimpanzees had become two distinct communities, the southern "Kahama community" and the original "Kasakela community." When the males of the two communities saw one another they made aggressive displays toward one another, then retreated back to their own territories.

During the third year of separation a patrol of six Kasakela adult male chimpanzees brutally attacked a young male from the Kahama community. This chimp was never seen again by the field staff and students working in the Kahama community's range and they believed he had died of his injuries. Over the next four years the researchers witnessed four more assaults of this kind. The third victim of these assaults was a former alpha chimpanzee of the Kasakela group named Goliath and known well by his assailants. One of the students who witnessed the assault stated that what shocked her most was the terrifying rage and hostility of the five aggressors. She felt they were "definitely trying to kill him." This chimp was a friend of Goodall and this was a tragic event for her.

After Goliath's death only three male Kahama chimps were left. The next victim was one of the three females left in the Kahama community, also well known to the Kasakela group. During the next year the rest of the adult Kahama males were attacked and killed. The last to be killed was a male called Sniff. Goodall tells it this way:

> Sniff was brutally murdered like the others. Hunted
> down, attacked and left incapacitated, bleeding from
> innumerable wounds and with a broken leg. Once again
> we all went out to search for him; once again we failed
> to locate the place where he had crept away to die. His
> passing marked the end of the Kahama community.

In the concluding section of her book, Goodall describes the above episodes as "the Four Years War against the Kahama deserters, the liquidation of the rebel males who turned their backs on their longtime friends and tried to make it on their own." Her characterization of the chimpanzee's behavior as making war agrees with Russell's observations; but Russell goes a step further and concludes that this warlike behavior was displaced aggression which if unleashed within the community would have destroyed the fabric of the community. He believes such aggression arises from the overproduction of the male hormone testosterone, and that the same condition exists in the human species.

DEVELOPING STANDARDS OF BEHAVIOR

Considering that dominance hierarchies, rank, and status have existed in primates for over thirty million years and that chaos can result when there is no leader or alpha individual, it seems a good bet that from an evolutionary standpoint this type of society has been selected for its survival value. Reconciliation, moralistic aggression, and revenge also seem to benefit a species by keeping its members in the group and persuading them to give as much as they take. However, like all systems, it may also have its drawbacks. The various above studies have provided some examples.

For one, the drive for dominance and status can become so consuming that individuals miss opportunities to mate and procreate; this can eliminate their genes from the gene pool of the species and important traits could be lost. In addition, moralistic aggression and revenge can be overdone and lead to warlike behavior, which has the potential to eliminate the attackers as well as the attacked. It also has the potential to provide generation after generation the grounds for waging continual war.

Since humans share many similarities with chimpanzees with respect to the drive for status and dominance and with respect to moralistic aggression and revenge, it seems reasonable to conclude that the prototype of human nature can be found among primates, and especially in chimpanzees. In addition to status, dominance, moralistic aggression, and revenge, we humans have developed the ability to conceptualize ourselves and judge our own behavior as well as that of others. Thus we have developed a whole range of emotional states which coincide with our judgments. We feel embarrassed, ashamed, guilty, proud, empowered, high esteem, low esteem, great importance, little importance, worthiness, unworthiness, sinfulness, born again, fallen, risen, and a whole host of other feelings that come with our self-consciousness.

Is there any evolutionary benefit to conceptualizing and judging of ourselves, or have these abilities merely piggybacked on our bigger brains and our ability to abstract, conceptualize, and symbolize? This is a difficult question to answer, and probably a case can be made either way. Initially, I believed that our sense of self just happened to ride along with the accumulation of our symbolic powers. But now I see some benefits to us as a species-as well as some drawbacks.

In chimpanzee society things flow smoothly as long as the alpha male and his coalition hold up. They have to keep order, as it were, and keep individuals in their respective places. The alpha male tries to control the mating practices of his subordinates and intimidate those who try to step out of line. However, as De Waal showed, rules of reciprocity, protection of infants by their mothers and retaliation also come into play. To enforce these rules, individuals have to take action against others, just as the alpha male must do.

As societies grow larger, it becomes more and more difficult to monitor individual actions and enforce the rules that leaders prescribe and other members of the societies live by. And the less the actions of the members are monitored and controlled, the more the potential exists for uncontrolled aggression and chaos. This was demonstrated when there was no effective leader in the Gombe chimpanzee community. On the other hand, if individuals monitored and controlled themselves, even when no authority figure was watching, this would allow for a larger society in which rules were followed. Individual members would be able monitor and control themselves if they could judge their actions and themselves against some acknowledged standard. This state of affairs would be beneficial for the society as a whole and add to its survival value.

In addition, if individuals were able to adhere to agreed-upon standards by virtue of their ability to internalize those standards and then judge or monitor their own internal states, this would produce a more cohesive and loyal group. Breaking the rules would produce shame and guilt and an attempt at self-retribution rather than having to have the leader or alpha male come over and show disfavor or anger. This would simplify the leader's responsibilities and allow the group to become quite a bit larger than the size of chimpanzee groups of fifty or so individuals.

So, from an evolutionary perspective, self-consciousness and self-evaluation could definitely have survival value for a group. The more that individuals accepted and lived by social values and rules, the stronger the bond would be with the group and the more their own identities would depend on the group. As long as they remained with their group, their own identities would remain intact.

In order to provide a large group of people with the same set of social values and rules, some type of language has to be involved. Around 3300 B.C. the first known written language, using cuneiform script, appeared. However, paleontologist Richard Leakey believes that late Homo erectus, the group of that lived until 800,000 years ago, had language and were a primitive version of modern humans.[6] If he is right, these people could have had a sense of self similar to ours and an ability to conceptualize that allowed for the internalization of norms and self-monitoring. Homo sapiens or modern humans, came along more than 100,000 years ago, with larger brains than Homo erectus and probably united into larger groups as well. With clothing, fire, weapons, and ingenuity available, humans managed to occupy practically every square inch of the earth in almost every conceivable climate. This eventually led to large groups of people in different parts of the world and the development of different physical features, including different skin pigmentation. While the term "race" is used to describe difference in pigmentation and physical features, (i.e. white race, black race, yellow race etc.), Rod Caird, in his book *Ape Man*, contends that the term "race" has no validity when applied to humans. He states,

> Most biologists would not even use the word race. In the context of human diversity, it has no scientific meaning at all. In fact you can find 80 percent of the world's genetic variation in any single population. Biologically, all humans are the same species, and they can and do mingle and breed with one another freely, wherever they come from and whatever they look like.

Then, he goes on to discuss a characteristic of human beings that he judges in a very unfavorable light. He writes,

> That said, there are obvious physical differences between the people of the world. Some are black, some are white, some are yellow, and with these skin colors go a set of characteristic hair and facial features. For some reason humans like to endow these differences with great significance, to attach ideas of superiority to one appearance over another. This habit has led to great conflict, pain and destruction. Racism is one of the most negative manifestations of the working of the human brain.

This, of course, fits with my assertion that making judgments about ourselves and others is part and parcel of being human. What Caird is objecting to, I assume, are the grounds for the judgments people make. Yet he ends up making a judgment about humanity using as a basis an abstract potential of mankind. It is the same evaluation used by Leakey when he stated that "we should rejoice at so wondrous a product of evolution." So, why don't we?

Looking at chimpanzee societies through the eyes of Russell, Goodall, De Waal, and others it can be seen that (1) community or group survival depends upon a strong leader who forms coalitions with others; (2) the survival of offspring depends upon the protection of their mothers or other female caretakers; (3) family survival depends upon the bonds formed between family members and their tendency to protect each other; (4) group order and prevention of interpersonal conflict depend upon dominance and rank as a way of life and rules of conduct reinforced by both positive and negative interventions; (5) a community's foraging area and territory are protected against intruders by male scouting groups led by an alpha chimpanzee.

These characteristics appear to have survival value for the species as a whole, since children are protected, order is maintained, cohesiveness of the group is preserved, procreation can occur and the group's resources are protected.

Is there any reason to believe that these characteristics disappeared or became unnecessary in the evolutionary line from ape man to modern human? Children still needed protection, the group still needed leadership, and group cohesion would still have been a priority. What about different groups living near each other; did they no longer defend their foraging areas or their territories? Did they no longer care whether members left the group to form new groups of their own? Was a sense of fairness no longer a priority, or did fairness become even more important as brains got bigger and abstract reasoning became more pronounced?

From humankind's recorded history, which goes back more than 5,000 years, we know that human groups grew larger and larger and that battles continually raged between them. Tribes, cities, city-states, and nations all did battle with each other for territory, power, possessions, and glory. And they not only conquered but also enslaved each other. Dominance, status, and rank were not only important but took on a more intense nature, with death rather than intimidation being the new reinforcer.

Should we really believe that this started only at the time of recorded history, or maybe several thousand years earlier? The characteristics that have been passed down the primate evolutionary line to the chimpanzee, and their close parallel to our own characteristics, say otherwise. Undoubtedly, we have added complexity to these characteristics through our abilities to conceptualize ourselves, use language, and make abstract rules of conduct based on concepts of fairness, ownership, and social order.

STAND UP STRAIGHT, DON'T SLOUCH

How and why apes got up on two feet-bipedalism-as a dominant form of locomotion is still a controversial subject among paleontologists, anthropologists, and others. And it seems that until this issue is resolved, nobody can speculate with any degree of confidence about the nature of the ape-man community that goes back millions of years. The formerly held belief that our ancestors arose to walk on two feet in order to adjust to a savanna-type environment has been undermined by recent findings that many of our ancestors like , *Ardipithecus ramidus*, lived in forests and wooded areas, and were bipedal creatures[8]

Similarly, if the argument is put forward that our manual dexterity, which allowed early humans to make tools and weapons, was the driving evolutionary force for bipedalism, the counter argument is always made that no tools were found for a period of at least a million years after apes first walked on two feet. Therefore, making tools and weapons cannot be considered an important factor in bipedalism. This reasoning may be a little spurious, however since chipped stones may not have been the first tools or weapons used by ape-men. Consider, for example, that chimpanzees throw rocks, hurl and flail branches when displaying aggressively. Goodall even noted that some chimps were better rock throwers than others, and that some chimps dragged huge branches behind them in their displays. One chimp, Mike, even kicked tin cans to intimidate his rivals. If throwing rocks and swishing branches can intimidate rivals, what prevents these props from being used as weapons for protection or attacking? And if standing upright can make rock-throwing and branch-flailing more effective, why wouldn't selection for standing upright for longer periods of time have been involved?

The use of rocks for throwing, branches for swinging and legs for kicking could have made a huge difference in the survivability of a community of apes or ape-men. Slowly, another species of an ape-like creature could have arisen who stood on his feet longer and eventually remained erect. This creature could then throw rocks with greater speed and accuracy and swing branches with greater force and precision. It is unlikely that the rocks he threw or the branches he swung would have survived as artifacts like the stone tools of *Homo habilis* found a million or so years later.

Likewise, branches both large and small could have been used as tools to poke things, knock things over, pry things apart and stab at things. If this use was passed on to others in the community or used by a male scouting party, there would then be a community of apes or ape-men armed with branches and rocks. A creature could have been stoned or battered to death just as modern humans were in the past and still are today. Offspring who practiced these pursuits could have become quite adept at them, with evolutionary selection playing an important part in bone and muscle formation. Once creatures stood erect, perhaps kicking was also developed. This ape-man would have been more lethal in intra-group squabbles or in vying for leadership. Accuracy in weapon use and strategy may have become as important as strength.

If this scenario is correct then greater hand and finger dexterity complemented the larger and larger brains that followed. Strategic and cooperative use of tools and weapons would have meant greater chances of survival. This would have required bigger brains. At some point self-conceptualization became an important factor, and then obtaining and maintaining identity would have become a primary focus for our ancestors.

FAMILY AND CULTURAL CONNECTIONS

The importance of having and maintaining an identity is spelled out clearly by anthropologist Jack Weatherford when he writes about slavery in his book *Savages and Civilization*. He concludes that the subsequent adjustment of the Jews who were enslaved by the Egyptians and the Africans, who were enslaved by people in North and South America, depended on their ability to maintain their cultural identity.[9]

He writes about the Jews:

> The rulers of the cities began raids and campaigns
>
> primarily to seize such captives, who were herded back
>
> to work in the fields, mines, and quarries of the captors.
>
> Thus it was that the nomadic tribes of the Hebrews
>
> tending their flocks were captured and taken into
>
> slavery by the armies of the pharaoh as well as by the
>
> Babylonians. The history of the ancient Jews illustrates
>
> a persistent problem from the perspective of the slave
>
> holders: As long as a group of slaves continued to live
>
> together in its traditional kinship groups, speaking its

own language, worshipping its own god, and generally following its own culture and way of life, it posed a threat to its owners. As long as slaves maintained their culture and some remnants of their tribal social structure, they were not totally conquered or assimilated into their social position as mere slaves.

In discussing the African slave situation Weatherford points out that the tribal people of Africa had a social structure consisting of kinship networks which did not survive the passage to America where even nuclear families were separated. He describes the dilemma of the slaves.

Africans who came to America as Ibo, Yoruba, Hausa, Bambara, or Malinke tribesmen became simply blacks, slaves, or Negroes. They were shorn of their native identity and issued a generic one in its place.

He goes on to explain how this helped the slave owners and hurt the enslaved Africans.

This cultural disorientation had an important function for the slave traders and owners, in that it minimized the likelihood that groups of slaves would conspire to escape or revolt. If the slaves could not talk adequately with one another, and if they shared little common culture, they were much less likely to assist one another in escaping. This conscientious and methodical destruction of tribal African culture persisted at every stage of the slavery system.

He concludes,

> The Jews survived slavery with their tribal culture intact, and were gradually able to adapt this older culture to new circumstances, to transform it gradually from a tribal one to an urban one that proved viable in Europe, India, and America as much as in Israel. The African slaves who were brought to the Americas never had this opportunity. They did not survive slavery with an intact tribal culture and society; they survived it with a slave culture within which they had remnants of African words, stories, ceremonies, music, and dance. From this they had to develop their own cultural traditions and create for themselves a place in society.

This conclusion lends weight to the idea that the development of self-awareness and identity was an evolutionary change that had survival value for our species. However, one can also see the drawback to this as it provides another area of vulnerability. This can be understood if one goes back to the beginning of Chapter II to see how Anna was affected. The problem of maintaining identity can be likened to the problem of maintaining life and physical well-being. Based on evolution, there are processes and systems that help protect, preserve, and maintain all three. These processes and systems are the engine of the psychological immune system, which I shall discuss in the next chapter.

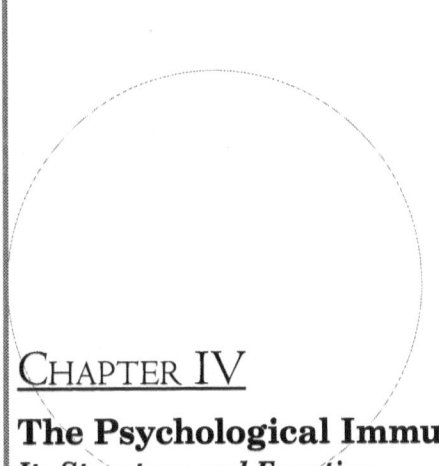

Chapter IV

The Psychological Immune System
Its Structure and Function

GENETIC PROGRAMMING

The psychological immune system (Psy-IS), like the biological immune system, is an outgrowth of the genetically programmed survival mechanisms that are built ("hard-wired") into all life forms. The system works to protect, preserve, and enhance (1) our life and physical well-being, (2) our sense of self and identity, and (3) our property and possessions. While property and possessions can be protected as unique entities they can also be intertwined with the protection of our lives, like our tools and weapons, and can be the products of our creative self, like intellectual property. Therefore, at times, the protection of our life and physical well-being is tied closely to our property and possessions and the protection of our sense of self and identity includes our artistic creations and intellectual property.

The Psy-IS directs us to attend to those aspects of our environment that are perceived as relevant to our lives, physical well-being, property/possessions, sense of self and identity. Thus we react more rapidly and forcefully to those stimuli we perceive as threatening and dangerous or beneficial and protective. In essence, the Psy-IS is an alerting and emotionally reactive system that makes use of our senses, our ability to discriminate between helpful, harmful and neutral things, our memory, and our conceptual ability, which includes our imagination and power to plan ahead. This gives us the ability of attending to both the dangerous and the life-saving or life-enhancing parts of our world and to formulate plans of action.

To take an example, when my son was about six years old he came to me one morning and said ,"Dad, I'd like to talk to you." Even though I was busy in the kitchen, I came over to the dining room table and said, "Sure, have a seat and we can talk." He proceeded to sit down next to me and then stated in a hesitant but pointed manner, "Dad, I've been thinking about moving next door."

To put it mildly, this came as a shock to me, since I thought I was doing a pretty good job as a father and had no idea that this was rolling around in my son's head. However, I was also very curious about the reason for this sudden urge, so I went along by saying, "Gee, I'm sorry to hear that. Is there a reason for you wanting to go next door?" What came out startled me even more. He said, "Well dad, you know that you're the smallest dad in the world."

This brought a defensive posture on my part, and I remarked, "I admit I'm small (I was about 5 ft 6 inches tall but have shrunk since then), but I don't think I'm the smallest dad in the world. Anyway, what does that have to do with anything?"

He continued along unhesitatingly, "Well, I've been wondering, if a burglar came in through the window, could you do anything about it?"

This really threw me off guard, and I answered as honestly as I could, something to the effect that I wasn't sure, but I would do the best I could. I then asked my son why he wanted to move next door. He said, "Well Ron, the man next door, is a lot bigger, and I would feel a lot safer there. " It was of course true that our next door neighbor was about six feet, two inches tall, so my son's perceptions were pretty accurate. He apparently felt safe talking to me, but not living with me.

Knowing pretty much how the situation was going to end, I told him that he could go next door and check with the neighbors to see if they were willing to take him in. He said he would think about it some more. The next day he informed me that he had thought it over and decided to stay with me. I told him I was very happy with his decision because I would be very sad if he moved away. He never brought this subject up again and I guess resolved in his mind that the safety factor was one consideration but not the only important one. This fits in well with the theme of the Psy-IS.

THE PSYCHOLOGICAL IMMUNE SYSTEM VS THE BIOLOGICAL IMMUNE SYSTEM

This story demonstrates that we, even as children, are constantly on the alert regarding our safety even if it isn't apparent to others who are close to us. In this regard the Psy-IS is no different from the biological immune system, which is always on the alert without our being aware of it. In fact, the Psy-IS emulates the biological immune system in many ways:

* Both have the goal-directed job of protecting, preserving, and enhancing our life and physical well-being.

* Both systems have to recognize and discriminate between helpful and harmful elements that confront us daily.

* Both systems must have some way of dealing with the harmful elements we encounter.

* Both systems make use of innate or nonspecific strategies as well as acquired specific means of defense.

* Both systems depend upon a homeostatic process that uses feedback mechanisms to stoke the defensive procedures up to a very high level when necessary and then return them to a neutral or non combative level when a threat has passed.

* Both systems depend upon memory of previous encounters with dangerous elements in order to respond more rapidly and forcefully the second time around.

* In addition, both systems can produce a deficient response, overreact to a non-serious threat, or turn on the individual they are supposed to protect. Overall, however, they help heal the body when it is injured. Both systems do quite a job!

BECOMING AROUSED

In these ways, the Psy-IS acts as a filter to screen the emotional meaning that everyday activities, events, relationships, and confrontations have for us. It does this through emotional messages and feelings that we consciously perceive and react to and emotions of which we are partially or unaware of but which also produce reactions. This type of system is well documented in *The Emotional Brain* by Joseph LeDoux, a neuroscientist at New York University.[1] When confronted by danger we almost instantaneously feel fear, anxiety, apprehension, and psychic arousal.

Sometimes we are not consciously aware of the danger until we are alerted by our feelings. For example: have you ever felt creepy and then noticed that someone was staring at you? Have you ever jumped when you heard a noise in the bushes near your home? Have you ever felt frightened when you heard a loud noise and it put you on alert, as though you were a radio antenna picking up remote signals ? Do you ever pick up messages from the faces of other people and stay out of their way when they had certain expressions? Have you ever felt inadequate around people you felt were more intelligent, more talented, or more attractive and didn't quite know how to act? If you answered "yes" to any of these questions you are not alone. It just means that your psychological immune system is doing its job and making you aware of the results. It allows you to evaluate your reactions and produce additional emotional responses such as shame, pride, disgust, determination to react differently the next time around, or self-acceptance. Thus we have a reaction to a situation and then an evaluative reaction to our reaction. We seem to constantly second-guess ourselves in our striving to make things better than before. This is the enhancing nature of the system.

Another important characteristic of the Psy-IS is that in addition to protecting, preserving, and enhancing our life and physical well-being, our property and possessions, and our sense of self or identity , we project this protective net to other individuals and groups we love, are bonded to, or with whom we identify. This makes good evolutionary sense, since we take so long in reaching maturity and need this protective net around us until we can go forth on our own. Families, clans, tribes, and nations also depend on this safety net when they are under attack and need to be defended by lots of group members. Of course, we are not the only species that displays this characteristic. For example, bears are most dangerous when their cubs are around; wolf packs act almost as one entity; lion prides defend their territory and each other; and the leader of a troop of chimpanzees depends on his coalition buddies to help him out when the going gets tough. So, although we have a saying that it's every man for himself, this is not exactly true. We also tend to be our brothers' keepers.

COMPOSITION OF THE PSYCHOLOGICAL IMMUNE SYSTEM

The psychological immune system, as I see it, is composed of six components that are regulated by six principles. Three apply to ourselves, and three apply to the people and groups we love, are bonded to or identify with. They are as follows:

1. The Psy-IS protects, preserves, and enhances (ppe) the life (LF) and physical well-being (WB) of ourselves (Us). In abbreviated form, the first principlebecomes: Psy-IS ppe (LF/WB) : Us

2. The Psy-IS protects, preserves, and enhances the life and physical well-being of the people and groups we love, are bonded to, or identify with (O>lv). In abbreviated form, the second principle becomes : Psy-IS ppe (LF/WB) : O>lv

3. The Psy-IS protects, preserves, and enhances the property (PT) and possessions (PS) of ourselves. In abbreviated form: Psy-IS ppe (PT/PS) : Us

4. The Psy-IS protects, preserves, and enhances the property and possessions (PT/PS) of the people and groups we love, are bonded to, or identify with. In abbreviatedform: Psy-IS ppe (PT/PS) : O>lv

5. The Psy-IS protects, preserves, and enhances the sense of self (SOS) and identity (IDT) of ourselves. In abbreviated form: Psy-IS ppe (SOS/IDT) : Us

6. The Psy-IS protects, preserves, and enhances the sense of self and identity (SOS/IDT) of the people and groups we love, are bonded to, or identify with. In abbreviated form: Psy-IS ppe (SOS/IDT) : O>lv

Putting all six principles and their components together in abbreviated form, we have:

1. Psy-IS ppe (LF/WB) : Us

2. Psy-IS ppe (LF/WB): O>lv

3. Psy-IS ppe (PT/PS): Us

4. Psy-IS ppe (PT/PS): O>lv

5. Psy-IS ppe (SOS/IDT): Us

6. Psy-IS ppe (SOS/IDT): O>lv

These six principles describe the components, nature, and function of the psychological immune system. What remains to be spelled out are the ways in which these principles manifest themselves in our daily lives, how they interact with each other, how they explain seemingly contradictory results of destruction rather than protection, what permutations and combinations result from using a six principle model, and what predictions can be made that might be testable in the future if someone were inclined to do so. This is what the book will attempt to do.

THE PRINCIPLES IN OPERATION:
LIFE AND PHYSICAL WELL-BEING

1. The psychological immune system protects, preserves, and enhances the life and physical well-being of ourselves.

2. The psychological immune system protects, preserves, and enhances the life and physical well-being of the people and groups we love, are bonded to or identify with.

The first two principles go together because they both deal with our life and the lives of people we are close to. To protect and preserve our life and physical well-being requires the coordination of many of our systems, including the nervous, endocrine, pulmonary, and cardiovascular systems. These, in turn, affect our musculo-skeletal system, which must take some action to keeps us in one piece.

This coordination has developed over millions of years and if it didn't exist we wouldn't be around to talk about it. Under stress, threats, and danger we have to get revved up so that we have the speed, stamina, and dexterity to meet the challenges facing us. This comes about because our senses trigger both conscious and unconscious emotional reactions in various areas of our brains, which in turn send signals to other parts of our brains that turn on the endocrine system and the sympathetic nervous system. These then activate our cardiovascular and musculo-skeletal systems. We end up, hopefully, making the right moves and the right   decisions to meet the threats and dangers that confront us or the people we love.

Just like the biological immune system, the whole process gets started when a threatening stimulus is recognized. With the Psy-IS it can be a spider or a snake, another person, a loud unexpected noise, a lightning flash, the loss of our brakes while driving, a scream from our house or apartment, a funnel cloud on the horizon, the loss of our purse or wallet or our child not coming home when expected.

I once had such a scare. When my daughter was about sixteen years old and didn't arrive when expected, at her girlfriend's house in Los Angeles after a Greyhound bus ride and another local bus ride, I was a bit nervous. I called the L.A. police department's downtown division which transferred me another division which polices the bus terminal, and I kept getting cut off so that I couldn't even make an intelligent report. After the third or forth attempt, my anxiety level was off the chart and my mind was racing, swinging back and forth between the worst scenarios and some innocuous mishap. A call from my daughter two hours later finally set my mind at ease, but an experience like that can certainly get your heart racing!

EMOTIONS GRAB OUR ATTENTION

Some of the stimuli that frighten us or cause anxiety are remnants from our evolutionary past, like spiders, snakes, and darkness, but most are probably learned from our parents, peers, and our own past experiences. But one thing is for sure: once a threat is perceived emotional reactions quickly follow, and this occupies our total attention. There is not much room for minor concerns, reading material, conversations about other subjects, or energy to concentrate on much of anything else. If you're occupied with stressful events while you are in school, you're not going to concentrate on your schoolwork very well.

Continued stress pushes us from occupation to preoccupation with the stressor. Preoccupation with a situation that has not been resolved yet is called worry. While unpleasant, it lets us know that we still have things to do, plans to make, or questions to ask of ourselves and others. It is not easy to let go of worry. Well-intentioned people who say, "Don't worry so much," are the same people who tell you, "Don't take things personally." Our emotional responses are not easily put aside by rational thoughts or the advice of others. While overreaction is possible, our emotions drive the thinking, planning, and action that have helped us survive and without which we couldn't function effectively.[2]

As parents have known throughout the ages, young children can be frightened by many different things: darkness, noises, people in costume (Chuck E. Cheese did a number on my grandson for many years), being left alone, and angry voices. Children also develop fear of imaginary figures like ghosts, goblins, witches, vampires, and giants. To a child all adults may look like giants! Since their imaginations can trigger the same emotional responses as real threats do, children need to practice and develop the ability to discriminate between real danger and imaginary ones.

They depend on their parents and other family members to help them with this task. That is one reason evolution has directed our Psy-IS to also focus on the people we love and are bonded with as well as on ourselves. Unfortunately, children often confuse real and imagined threats, and readily make up scary stories. Parents must figure out which is which, and this is not an easy job.

For example, a child says someone came into her room at night and stared at her. Is she imagining this, or did it really happen? A child says someone came into his room, got into bed with him, and touched him: imagination, or reality? A child says her stepfather came into her room and fondled her: real or not real? A child tells you tales of weird things that happened at preschool. Is her imagination working overtime? If you believe the child, you get in touch with the police or children's protective services and let them investigate. They can't always tell either, and when and if the case comes to trial, even the judge or jury may not be able to tell.

Of course, it's not only children who have good imaginations. Many adults can also weave a good tale, from being kidnapped by space aliens to communicating with the dead. The world has its share of tall tales. Many adults may believe what they say but others are con artists trying to take advantage of gullible people. Hustling others can be a livelihood. As with children, it isn't always easy to distinguish truth from fiction.

One of the reasons it is difficult to know whether a child is being frightened by a real or imaginary event is that children often use play and make-believe to better understand their world.

They play out their fears in order to conquer them. They try on many different roles and play out many different scenarios. This is a coping strategy of the psychological immune system.

Some time ago, for example, when my grandson, Jacob, was five years old, he came running into my house with a friend of his and said in a very emotional voice, "Papa," (the name he called me) "Eric just crashed my Jeep into a tree and it caught on fire." Now, I knew that Jacob and his friends had used the battery-operated Jeep many times during the past year, and nothing like that had ever happened before, so I doubted his story. I looked him squarely in the eyes and said, "Look, this is a very serious matter and nothing to play around with. So you'd better not be telling me a story!" Jacob eyeballed me back and insisted, "I'm not kidding! The jeep got crashed and it's on fire!" His friend backed up the story of the Jeep being on fire, but denied that he had crashed it into a tree. The continued intensity of their emotions, which I gleaned from their speech and body language, finally convinced me that my grandson was telling the truth, so I ran outside the house and followed them around the corner to the street west of the house. Sure enough, about twenty-five yards up the street I saw the jeep next to a large tree, and the front of it was on fire. I managed to put the fire out and pushed the Jeep back to the house. I removed the battery, the burnt wires, and most of the burnt plastic. The Jeep cooled off in about fifteen minutes.

What was fascinating, however, were the ways my grandson and his friend played out the Jeep being in a wreck, turning over, catching fire, and injuring both of them. This playing out continued for the next two hours. Jacob told his parents all about the mishap when they came to pick him up, and he talked about the event, with lots of emotion, for the next two weeks. A year later, he still remembered it well and seemed to have more of an understanding of the emotional impact a car wreck has on people. As the saying goes, experience is the best teacher. Perhaps we should add the word "emotional" to "experience" to make the saying fit the facts better. Emotional experiences stay with us a lot longer than non-emotional ones, and some that have been buried for a long time can be revived by stresses that may not even be related to the original event.[3]

THE POWER OF BELIEF

Whereas my grandson experienced emotional arousal when he saw the Jeep on fire, I experienced emotional arousal when he told me about it. I had to convince myself that what I heard was real and not imaginary before I sprang into action. Words, of course, can produce the same intense emotional reaction as seeing something happen if the individual believes the word to be truthful. Take someone shouting "fire" in a theater. If you believe there is a fire, you're going to experience the same intense emotional reaction you would if you actually saw the fire yourself. If an individual tells you there is someone down the street with a gun coming to get you and you believe it, you will experience the same emotional reaction you would if you saw the person yourself. Thus, our belief system can be a trigger to intense emotions.

For instance, the Salteux branch of the Ojibway Indians, who live in Manitoba, Canada, believe that any physical ailment like a headache, a raspy throat, or an upset stomach is a penalty for "bad conduct." Misconduct can include insults, failure to share with others, selfish acts, cruel acts and even injuring or killing someone. Thus, such ailments produce intense anxiety, for they are expected to progress into major illnesses that could become life-threatening. Public confession of one's bad conduct is the only way the Salteux believe they can head this off. As a person's confession spreads through the tribe children learn what kind of conduct is bad and needs to be avoided. Since there is no council or court system to pass judgment, anxiety plays the part of maintaining proper conduct.[4]

In our western society, if individuals react to physical distress with more anxiety than seems warranted because they believe the distress to be caused by serious or life-threatening problems that have no medical basis, we would say they suffer from a panic or anxiety disorder. In any case, belief can be a potent trigger for anxiety. The biological immune system's overreaction to non threatening stimuli is called an allergic reaction. Perhaps the psychological immune system's overreaction should be called an emotional or psychological allergic reaction.

In order to protect, preserve, and enhance our lives and the lives of those we love, the Psy-IS depends upon both "innate" or inborn emotional reactions and "acquired"or learned reactions. This resembles the processes used by the biological immune system to protect life. But whereas the biological immune system relies strictly on a cause-and-effect physical model, the Psy-IS makes use of our symbolic and conceptual abilities. In effect, we are always trying to make sense of the world by understanding our emotional reactions to it. When the Psy-IS is confronted by the prospect of being unable to protect both our own life and that of someone we love, a choice has to be made, and this can tear at the very fabric of the system.

Saving one's own life versus sacrificing one's life for a loved one is a dilemma that has shadowed humanity for eons. This is the kind of issue that we will examined in the next chapter along with human behavior that seems to contradict the principles of the Psy-IS. For now, let us continue our exploration of the rest of the principles and components of the Psy-IS.

PROPERTY AND POSSESSIONS

3. The psychological immune system protects, preserves and/or enhances the property and possessions of ourselves.

4. The psychological immune system protects, preserves and/or enhances the property and possessions of those we love.

In a capitalistic system in which private property abounds and there is enough money to buy whatever one wants or needs, these two principles go a long way toward explaining some of our tenacious behavior toward our property and possessions and why so many laws pertain to owning, selling, buying, and trading property. But how about non-capitalistic systems, and how about primitive man? Do these same principles also apply to them?

We know that our ancestors made tools from stone some two million years ago and that art objects and paintings have been uncovered from at least 30,000 years ago. We also know that individuals were buried with adornments at least 20,000 years ago. For example, in Russia, archeologists uncovered four well preserved burials-of a man, a woman, and two adolescent children-dated between 25,000 and 20,000 years ago. The man was buried together with blades of ivory, and wore a headband and necklaces made up of mammoth ivory beads. The adolescent children were buried head to head along with ivory beads, rings, ornaments, the teeth of arctic fox, and weapons including spears, spear-throwers, and daggers.[5]

Monuments, such as the monoliths at Stonehenge in England and the pyramids in Egypt date back to some 4,000 years ago. In Sumer, a land in the Near East where written language began over 5,000 years ago, wheeled vehicles, wheel-made pottery, sailboats and animal-drawn plows were written about as were conflicts over land and water rights.[6] The existence of tools, art objects, and monuments thousands of years old certainly suggests that the value of these and other items clearly registered in the mind of humans. Tools that ensured survival and art objects that adorned the body to enhance attractiveness and identity would certainly be protected and preserved. Monuments that represented the pride and identity of their societies also would receive special protection, and most likely so did land and water rights as well.

Protection of land or territory goes back a long way. It was, and still is, practiced by our closest living relatives, the chimpanzees. Both behavioral biologist Richard D. Estes and Jane Goodall, who studied the Gombe chimps for thirty years, have written books that support this conclusion.[7,8] Chimps who stray into the territory of neighboring groups are fair game for being attacked and severely injured or killed.

This phenomenon has been most pronounced in Gabon, Africa, where the logging of portions of the tropical rain forests has frightened the chimp inhabitants into the territory of other chimps. As a result, according to field biologist Lee White of the Wildlife Conservation Society, warfare has broken out between the different chimp communities, and many deaths have occurred. In fact White estimates that about 30,000 chimps have been killed in this manner, during 1999 alone![9]

Closer to home, I often noticed that my late German Shepherd and my mixed-breed dog were quite territorial when we went camping. People and other dogs who got too close to our van or our campsite were notified quite vigorously that they were intruding. It took a lot of reassuring to convince the dogs that everything was all right and they could relax. Some dogs protect food, toys, territory, and human family members, according to Jacque L. Schultz , Director of Special Projects, ASPCA Animal Sciences. She claims that many breeds, including cocker spaniels and Labrador retrievers, put on "ferocious displays

over toys and chewies resulting in punishing bites to hands and faces"
of people who are unaware of the dogs' protective tendencies.[10]

BATTLING FOR PROPERTY

The history of humanity has also been a saga of wars between
different tribes, nation-states, and empires over maintaining or
expanding their territories. Individual private property rights
were written about by Sumarian scribes some 4,000 years ago.[11]
Conflicts and fights over personal property, land ownership, and
property rights-both material and intellectual-were still going
strong in the twentieth century, and it doesn't look like there
will be any letup in the twenty-first century or beyond. In the
1990s, warring factions competed for control over administrative
institutions and territory in Afghanistan, Angola, Azerbaijan,
Cambodia, Croatia, the Congo, Iraq, Liberia, and Indonesia, to
name a few.[12, 13]

In 1999, the heaviest fighting since the war of 1971 resumed
between India and Pakistan over the disputed territory of
Kashmir.[14] Land, of course, is important not only to nations
but also to companies that use the land to extract products
such as oil and minerals. Sometimes, this sets up competition
for the same land, and very emotional confrontations can ensue.
For example, the U'wa tribe in Colombia has been trying to
prevent the Occidental Petroleum Company from drilling for
oil on land that they claim is part of their ancestral territory.
Occidental Petroleum, spent $12 million on seismic tests in
hopes of drilling in the remote region of the U'wa Indians,

and had applied for a drilling permit from the Colombian government. The U'wa cause was joined by three Americans: Terence Freitas, a biologist from the Los Angeles area; Ingrid Washinawatok, an Indian rights advocate from the Menominee Reservation in Keshena, Wisconsin; and Lahe'ena'e Gay, director of the Hawaii-based Pacific Cultural Conservancy International. During the week before the February 26, 1999, deadline for the decision on Occidental's permit, Freitas tried to get the organization Amazon Watch to send letters to the Colombian ministry on behalf of the U'wa tribe. In addition he, Wahinawatok, and Gay helped the tribe establish bilingual schools on its reserve.

The meeting between Los Angeles-based Occidental Petroleum Corporation and the U'wa tribal president, Robert Cobaria, in 1997 had failed to resolve the differences between the two. After Freitas joined the U'wa cause, he received death threats on his answering machine, something to the effect, "back off or die." These threats apparently reflected the intensity with which someone wanted Occidental to drill for oil on the contested land, because in early March 1999 the bodies of all three Americans were found in a cow pasture blindfolded and bound at their wrists. Four bullet holes were found in each woman, and six in Terry Freitas.[15]

HOLDING ON TO POSSESSIONS

Competition for possessions and articles of interest seems to start at a very early age. One can notice children as young as eighteen months taking possession of objects, holding on to these objects for dear life, and fighting with other children over them. Parents, day care workers, and teachers spend an inordinate amount of time settling disputes between children about what belongs to whom and acting as judge and jury to decide who is being fair and who is being selfish in sharing toys with others. Children seem to be keenly aware of who has a bigger toy, who is allowed to spend more time with a favored toy, and who is hogging certain toys.

This issue sprang to life when I took my grandson to a four-acre cornfield maze in July of '99 that we and others paid to find our way through. When we arrived we joined another family of three other children aged four through ten, and their parents. Before we entered the maze we were given a short lecture on the rules, like no picking the corn and no running; some hints about finding our way out by looking for clues of colored ribbon and mailboxes containing sections of a map; and a flag on top of a long pole that each family was supposed to carry through the maze. This last item was not a good idea for the family of four children because the flag and flagpole could not be split four ways and it immediately became a source of contention. Despite the best efforts of the adults, there was constant grabbing, shoving, hitting, crying and shouts of "my turn." The urge to possess this particular object came from both the desire to handle a new "toy" and the desire to hold status within the family. Thus, in addition to utilitarian value, objects can possess symbolic value, and this adds another dimension to the emotional urge to protect, preserve, and enhance property and possessions. Our biological immune system reacts to the antigenic properties of microorganisms but, as far as anyone knows, not to any symbolic properties of those organisms. Think of the confusion and theoretical upheaval that would be generated if the immune system had to figure out whether a virus or bacteria was making a symbolic overture or a real attack.

As previously mentioned when discussing the first two principles, the Psy-IS sometimes has the the unenviable task of choosing between protecting and preserving one component of the system over another, such as one's own life or the life of a loved one. The same dilemma can befall the Psy-IS in respect protecting your property and possessions or of those of someone you love, are bonded to, or identify with. When a fire breaks out, do you save your coin collection or photo albums first or your mate's stamp collection. To complicate matters even more, you may feel pressure to run back into the burning house and save a very precious heirloom. This creates a conflict between the Psy-IS's mandate to protect and preserve your life and the mandate to protect and preserve your property and possessions. Nations face this same dilemma when governments consider whether the lives of its soldiers are worth the territory it wants to defend or acquire. As comedian Jack Benny said, after a shortpause, when a robber demanded "Your money or your life"... "I'm thinking, I'm thinking!"

SENSE OF SELF AND IDENTITY

This brings me to the last two principles of the psychological immune system, namely:

5. The psychological immune system protects, preserves and/or enhances our sense of self and identity.

6. The psychological immune system protects, preserves and/or enhances the sense of self and identity of those we love, are bonded to or identify with.

Chapter II looked at how we continually evaluate and monitor our worth and sense of self. These evaluations, together with our familial, social, ethnic, religious, professional, and national affiliations make up our identity. Our psychological immune system acts as a filter for the experiences we encounter in our daily lives. It reacts with emotion when we encounter situations or events that we perceive as having very negative or very positive effects on our sense of self or our identity. This also holds for the sense of self and identity of those persons we are close to. The intensity of our emotions serves as a yardstick to measure how much impact our experiences have on our sense of self and/or our identity.

We have various ways of protecting and preserving as well as enhancing our sense of self and identity. At times, we seem to both protect and enhance at the same time. For example, when we demean or scapegoat others, we do so in order to protect our own sense of self and we feel enhanced in our superiority to others.

Perhaps the following story will bring out some of these points more clearly. I, another psychologist and a teacher-all from the Mental Health Department-were discussing with a third-grade class the kind of problems they encountered in their class. One brave girl volunteered that John, one of the boys in the class, was always pushing and hitting people. He would push his way to the front of the line and dared anyone to stop him. After this revelation, other members of the class joined in and spoke of the punishments they had endured at the hands of John. The class was unanimous in condemning John's behavior, and they volunteered that no matter what they tried it seemed to do no good. He was a bully, and he was determined to stay a bully.

They revealed that John had been warned that he was about to be thrown out of school, but even that was not enough to curb his behavior. Their teacher verified the students' remarks and said that she and the school administrators had tried everything, and John was indeed in peril of being expelled from school. She went on to say that he not only hits the kids in his class, but also gets into fights with kids in other classes during recess.

I wrote on the blackboard that the problem could be defined as John's need to be a bully, and that he wanted to show everybody how tough he was. This was so important to his sense of self that he was willing to risk getting expelled from school in order to maintain his tough image. Getting into fights with other students was his way of showing how tough he was. I asked the class if this defined the problem clearly and they agreed. Then I went over to John and asked him if what the class had said about his behavior was true, and whether the core of the problem was his need to show how tough he was by fighting, hitting, and pushing other students around.

John admitted that he hits other students sometimes, but not as often as they were saying. He felt that they were exaggerating and they egg him on by teasing and daring him. I asked John if he liked to fight, and he said, "No I don't like fighting." I then asked him why he got into so many fights, and he said that the other students in the class "set him up." I asked him to explain what he meant by that. He went on to state that during recess the kids in his class would go up to the kids in other classes and say that they had the toughest kid of the school in their class, and that he could whip any kid in the other class. The other kids, of course, maintained that this wasn't true, and they told the toughest kid in their class that John said he could kick his behind. The kids then gathered around and goaded the two kids into a fight. John said he hated having to fight, but he couldn't back away and have others believe he was a "sissy."

This was quite a mouthful from John, and it took the teacher and us mental health consultants by surprise. So we asked the other students if what John said was factual. After hemming and hawing for a while they admitted that they bragged to other classes about how tough John was, and that fights did result from this. However, they were quick to add that they thought John liked to fight and they were surprised and shocked to hear John say that he didn't. After hearing all this I went back to the blackboard and wrote that part of the problem was that they liked to watch John fight the kids in other classes and took pride in his aggressiveness and toughness but complained when he turned his aggressiveness on them.

Since John didn't want to fight and the other students didn't want John to bully them, it was pretty easy to get John and his classmates to work out a compromise. He would stop bullying them if they would stop bragging about his toughness and setting up fights at recess. We told the class that we would return in two weeks to see how things were. When we came back two weeks later, we learned from the teacher and the students that everything was going great and that John had been accepted into the class as a friend and not as a bully. We asked John how he felt about the change, and he admitted he liked it a lot better, but he wondered if we could help him out with the problem of his older brother always hitting him and calling him a sissy. This remark made John's behavior more understandable.

I thought to myself that it was a shame nobody had gone into John's brother's class and helped him see the role aggression plays in covering up a fear of being seen as weak or cowardly and enhancing one's sense of self at the expense of others. And then again, it is probably a shame that nobody was able to point out this kind of protective mechanism to John's father, because we now know that patterns of behavior are passed down from generation to generation. Although protecting one's sense of self and identity is inborn, the methods used are learned from one's family and associates.

It is interesting to consider how the other members of the class singled out John as the problem and ignored their own contribution to the problem. They were intimidated by his behavior toward them, but also took pride in the fact that he represented their class's toughness in competition with other classes. They acted as fight managers, as it were, and were also the cheering crowd. They rationalized away their behavior and convinced themselves they were doing nothing wrong. In effect, they took the high moral ground. It was not until John said he didn't like to fight that they realized they were acting as fight managers without the fighter's consent.

Another point brought out by the episode of the third-grade class is how easily we become part of the groups in which we spend time and then try to protect, preserve, and enhance the group as we do our own sense of self and identity. Our ability to conceptualize, think and talk about the group even when we are not with the group makes our connection more personally meaningful. Thus, John's classmates had to weigh their desire to enhance their own class identity through his toughness against their desire to protect their physical well-being. Without class problems being clarified there is little chance for the students to find workable solutions, so the burden to solve interpersonal problems falls on the teacher and administration. To me, uncovering the roots of school interpersonal problems and getting the student to solve them is just as or more important than learning academic subjects.

THE SHAPING OF OUR IDENTITY

The teacher plays an important role in defining her or his class, and more than likely compares her or his class to other classes of the same grade level. The teacher may not be in competition with the other classes, but can't help feeling proud when children in her class achieve and disappointed when they do not. Children are pretty good at picking up the teacher's expectations and feelings about the class. How important the opinions of teachers are to their children's sense of self can be seen in the famous experiment in prejudice by third-grade teacher Jane Elliot.

Elliot randomly designated brown-eyed children as superior to blue-eyed children. She gave the brown-eyed children special privileges and had the blue-eyed children obey stricter rules because they were "inferior." Within a day, the blue-eyed children began to do more poorly in their schoolwork. They also became more depressed, sullen, and angry and described themselves as "sad," "bad," "stupid," and "mean." In the meantime, the brown-eyed students became nasty, vicious third graders. They refused to play with their former friends and accused them of stealing things. When Elliot reversed things the next day and proclaimed that she had made a mistake and, in reality, blue-eyed children were superior to brown-eyed children, the same results ensued as the previous day but in reverse.[16]

Just as our bodies develop and grow from infancy to adulthood, our sense of self and identity do likewise. But although the body stops growing as we reach adulthood, our sense of self and identity do not stop. We continue to evaluate, judge and work on ourselves until our death. Thus, our psychological immune system has to maintain an awareness of who we are in order to know what to protect, preserve, and enhance. Our thoughts, our feelings, our emotions, and our actions provide the feedback necessary to accomplish this task.

Psychiatrist Donald L. Nathanson, who studied the affect theory (which deals with our emotions) of psychologist Silvan S. Tomkins, is convinced that we evaluate our actions against a continuum along the shame/pride axis and that our sense of self comes from where we place ourselves along this axis. Our experiences of shame and pride and our evaluations are closely linked to the cultures in which we live.[17]

Nathanson would, most likely, explain the episode of John and his third-grade class and the brown-blue-eyed class experiment in terms of the shame and pride dichotomy. He theorizes that there are four ways in which we deal with our shame: we withdraw from the situation when we can't take the pain anymore; we attack ourselves, endure public humiliation, and become masochistic; we avoid the feeling and/or intensity of shame through various techniques; and we attack others by words and deeds.

MAKING CHOICES

Whatever techniques and strategies our Psy-IS uses to protect, preserve, and enhance our sense of self and our identity, it must do the same for our life and property. This is not an easy task, and many times our Psy-IS has to choose among the various options available. For example, I recall that when I was about nine or ten years old I was confronted by two teenage boys who wanted my money. The fear generated was based on the immediate evaluation that my life and physical well-being were in danger. I felt weak and helpless. I had ten cents to my name and needed it for bus fare to get home. If anger and humiliation were there, they were not strong enough to overcome my fear. My immediate reaction was to plead my case for letting me keep my dime for bus fare. They must have felt some pity for me, for they let me keep my money and allowed me to go to the bus stop. So, in this situation, my Psy-IS opted to protect and preserve my life and physical well-being at the expense of my pride and self-esteem. Examples of this kind are familiar to most people as they occur all throughout our lives and they will be explored more thoroughly in the coming chapters.

In the Eskimo culture, in the not too distant past, economic partnerships and social alliances between men were often formalized by sharing each other's wives for a short time. However, if a wife had sexual relations with another man without the approval of her husband, the offended husband had to take revenge on the other man, or he would live the rest of his life in shame. Many homicides resulted from this accepted way of behaving. In this case, protecting one's sense of self took priority over one's life and physical well-being. However, other outlets were also developed to protect, preserve, and enhance one's sense of self and identity without risking one's life. These included: buffeting (giving each other forceful blows until one man was felled); butting (opponents strike each other with their foreheads, and the one who gets upset first is derided by the onlookers); wrestling (done before the entire village with the winner gaining social status and esteem); and song duels (which consisted of lampoons, insults, and obscenities intended to humiliate one's opponent. The winner was the one who got applause after many verses, while the loser suffered humiliation and disapproval of the group).[18]

GROUP AFFILIATION

Preserving and enhancing one's sense of self and identity can become somewhat confusing to the Psy-IS when one becomes a part of many different groups, each with its own expectations, rituals, and loyalty requirements. For example, take the Indians from New York State who spoke various dialects of the Iroquoian language. The tribes all lived in protected villages along streams or lakes and inside the villages were rectangular longhouses, each occupied by an extended matrilineal family. Five tribes formed a union called the League of the Five Nations : the Mohawk, the Oneida, the Onondaga, the Cayuga, and the Seneca. Among the Iroquois, each individual was part of a nuclear family, which belonged to a household, which lived with other households in a longhouse, which constituted part of a clan, which belonged to a moiety, which made up a tribe, which in turn was part of the League of the Iroquois. Thus each individual had a multitude of sub-identities, which could make for a variable and confusing identity.[19]

The same variability and confusion can be witnessed in modern societies. Each person belongs to a *nuclear family*, which can be part of a larger *extended family*. The family is part of a *neighborhood,* which is part of a *city,* which in turn is a member of the *county* in a given *state or territory.* The state or territory makes up part of the *country.* Therefore, an individual named Zany can conceive of himself as a member of the Zantus family in the Zee street neighborhood within the city of Zoom, the county of Zanta, the state of California, and the country of the United States of America. If you met him on the street and asked him who he was he might say, "I'm Zany Zantus from the Zee street neighborhood, and I'm proud to be an American living in Zoom, California from the county Zanta, known for its zinc and its zinnias." If you were interviewing Zany you might ask him if he belonged to a religious group and what ethnic background he came from. He might say that he was a Zoroastrian and had a Persian ancestry. You might then enquire about his political affiliations, and he would tells you that he belonged to the Green Party and was an environmentalist through and through. He would go on to say that he was a marathon runner and coached his daughter Zelda's soccer team. How about his job or his profession? Well, he was a teacher of Zoology at Zanta Junior College.

So now what do we have? We have Zany Zantus the zoology teacher and Zoroastrian from the Zee street neighborhood who is married and is a father with a daughter, Zelda, and the coach of her soccer team. He has a Persian ancestry and is a marathon runner who belongs to the Green Party. He lives in the city of Zoom, in the county of Zanta, in the state of California, and is proud to be an American. While Zany has to put these all together, somehow, into an identity, we haven't even talked about his socioeconomic status, his military record, his artistic talents and interests, or any other group he is affiliated with.

What an individual finds most important for his identity and sense of self is quite an individual matter and hard to predict until the individual's sense of self and identity are threatened. This is so because adversity and struggle help a person define himself more clearly. Those parts that rise up to meet a challenge (or fail to meet a challenge) stand out more sharply in people's minds.

Like individuals, groups also develop identities. Members of the group get a feel for the group's identity over time, they bond with the group and their Psy-IS then strives to protect, preserve and enhance the group. This is called group loyalty. This was seen in John's third-grade class and applies to members of larger societies and nations as well. The individuals who become leaders or come to represent the groups protect the identities and reputations of their groups with the same-and sometimes greater- intensity than that with which they protect their own identities and reputations. Sometimes, in fact, members of the group rely almost totally on the group for their own identities and sense of self. Under these circumstances, members are willing to trade their own lives for the benefit of the group.

As we have seen, conflicts and wars pitting one group or nation against another have continued throughout the twentieth century. In fact, it was the bloodiest century in the history of mankind. The built-in intensity of the psychological immune system to eliminate threats to the life, property and identity of individuals and groups goes a long way in explaining these conflicts. This conclusion will be enlarged upon in the coming chapters.

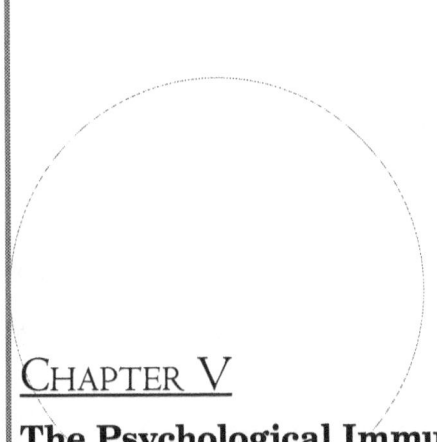

CHAPTER V

The Psychological Immune System In Action
Issues and Conflicts Addressed

FEAR AND PRIDE

Suppose you sat your infant on the floor and placed a new stuffed animal in front of him or her. You stand behind your infant and inflate a large balloon. As your infant reaches out to touch the stuffed animal, you stick a pin into the balloon so that it bursts with a loud noise. What do you guess would happen?

In 1920, such an experiment was conducted on an infant named Albert. In this case, the boy was exposed to a white rat instead of a stuffed animal and the loud noise was made by a gong. After seven trials, Albert became frightened by the mere sight of the white rat, without the loud noise. The association of a neutral object with something that creates fear until the neutral object creates the same fear reaction, is called fear conditioning.

It is difficult to undo the conditioned fear and it can spread to other objects that resemble the original neutral object. Albert's fear spread to other furry objects such as a rabbit, a dog, and even a Santa Claus mask, and his natural inclination was to avoid or run away from the feared objects once he saw them.[1]

Children do not necessarily have to see, hear, or touch what they become afraid of. By tapping into children's keen imagination, their fears can be unleashed by and hooked onto a variety of situations or objects. I still recall vividly the fear generated by teens regarding the "woods" around our neighborhood when I was a child. They spoke of "child-eating, half-man, half-apes" in the trees that they knew well and that would not attack us if the teens were with us. We just had to keep our heads down and never look up at the treetops. Sometimes, as we walked through the woods with the teens, the temptation arose to look up and see what was there, but I never did. I dared not go alone through those woods, for fear of my life. The fear was palpable whenever I rode or walked near those woods.

Stories told around the campfire can keep kids up all night listening for strange noises and can hold them close to their buddies, who are just as frightened. Movies and videos depend on children's fear reactions. When I was young, _The Clutching Hand_ was a weekly serial at the movies that came on the screen between the double - features. This hand would come out of the woodwork or walls in a house and grab people by the throat. It scared the bejeesus out of me, and when I got home I would stay away from the walls in the apartment for fear of being grabbed by that clutching hand.

It makes good evolutionary sense that early humans tried to avoid, animals, situations, or events that produced anxiety and fear. When our ancestors tamed fire, some half a million years ago,[2] they were more than likely happy that they could finally light up their caves and keep dangerous animals at bay. Our modern fear of the dark, the unknown, great heights, and slithering snakes may be left over from our ancestors. The above observations fit in well with the first principle of the psychological immune system, namely: that humans are genetically programmed to protect, preserve, and/or enhance their lives and physical well-being. In essence, it implies that people are programmed to avoid things that were experienced as dangerous or hurtful or were revealed by trusted others as dangerous or harmful. These are things that generate anxiety and fear.

What is harmful to children? What causes pain and distress? What produces anxiety and fear? By answering these questions we would come to know what children try to avoid, right? Definitely wrong! As strong as the program is to protect, preserve and/or enhance one's life and physical well-being, there is another built-in program that competes for expression. Below are two examples of what I'm talking about.

While at a museum my fourteen-month-old granddaughter, Sarah, encountered a skinned black bear hanging lengthwise over a wooden railing and watched as her seven-year-old brother rubbed the bear's fur. While holding on to my hand, she pulled me toward the bear and signaled for me to touch the fur, which I did. I could sense her desire to touch the fur as she held her hand near it but her fear prevented her from doing so. After repeating this little ritual of signaling me to touch the bear's fur and holding her hand near the fur but not touching it, we moved on to other exhibits. But, it was not long before she pulled me toward the skinned bear once more and reached out to touch its fur only to pull her hand away in fear once again. Although she persisted several more times toward the goal of touching the fur, she never gathered up enough courage to do so. Given such fear, one has to wonder why she was so persistent about going back time after time and raising her anxiety level instead of staying away and keeping her level of fear at a minimum.

This next example involves Sarah's brother, Jacob, when he was eighteen-months-old. While walking through J.C. Penny we spotted a life-sized stuffed lion that represented Simba in *The Lion King*. When we pointed out the lion to our grandson, he seemed a little taken aback and asked to be picked up and carried. My wife obliged and we started walking over to the stuffed animal. The closer we got the more anxious Jacob became, and he indicated by word and body language that he wanted to keep his distance from the lion. But when we had retreated to where we had started he urged my wife to take him back to look at the lion again from a closer perspective. As they approached the stuffed lion, Jacob reached out to touch it only to withdraw his hand in utter terror before it reached the lion. He continued this approach - avoidance behavior several more times before he finally summoned up enough courage to reach out and touch the lion. The thrill of victory resonated through his whole body, and as we were leaving the store he loudly and proudly announced to anyone coming toward us, "I touchy yion!, I touchy yion!" He repeated this mantra all the way home and triumphantly related to his parents the feat that he had just accomplished.

From the perspective of the psychological immune system, these two episodes can be seen as Sarah's and Jacob's attempts to protect and preserve their lives or physical well-being by distancing themselves from the menacing animals while at the same time being pushed by internal forces to preserve and enhance their sense of self or identity by engaging and attempting to touch the fearsome beasts, which Jacob finally succeeded in doing. How does such a young child summon enough courage to engage a feared object? And, for that matter, what inspires a toddler to get up and try again and again to walk after falling down numerous times and hurting him or herself? Why do youngsters get back on their bikes and skateboards after skinning their knees and elbows?

As I view the psychological immune system, the motivating force that challenges and overcomes the fear of injury is the genetic program to protect, preserve and/or enhance one's sense of self or identity, which manifests itself in pride of accomplishment and distress of failure. This program unfolds around nine months of age and, as the above examples show, is going strong by eighteen months of age.[3] Parents, siblings, and peers, of course, are the audience and cheering section that watches the drama of the conflict between safety and pride as it is played out in young children. So, trying to scare children about the hazards of certain types of behavior may have the opposite effect. It may engage their sense of pride in risk-taking and doing hazardous things in order to prove their worth to themselves and others. And getting away with things without getting caught can be a turn-on all by itself. Parents, teachers and educators should therefore consider the conflict between safety and pride before trying to use scare tactics. In fact, getting children to talk about this conflict would provide a good entree into their psyches and suggest ways to help them chart a safe course in handling this conflict.

The difference in personality traits among children-shyness, boldness, the degree of inhibition or the degree of maturity-can account for whether the safety or pride component will gain the upper hand in a given situation. But, Dr. Jerome Kagan concludes that despite the mistaken belief that personality is laid down in the first three years of life, children do not remain the same over the years, and the shy, inhibited youngster of today can become the bold, uninhibited adolescent of tomorrow and people have the capacity to change across their entire life span.[4,5]

THE PUSH TOWARD RISK-TAKING

Placing the emphasis on competition, which is so prevalent in western societies, has a tendency to add intensity to the conflict between safety and pride. By emphasizing individuality, toughness, and winning, society creates pressure to choose enhancement of one's sense of self over protection and preservation of one's physical well-being. Hence, risk-taking becomes a matter of choice that leads to a boost in self-esteem when successful. The end result is that the greater the risk, the greater the potential payoff in stature and self-enhancement. However, the greater the risk, the greater the possible harm to one's physical well-being. More and more individuals are trying skateboarding stunts, rock climbing, hang-gliding, snow boarding, mountain climbing and dirt biking, in which the risk of injury becomes a "turn- on." The X Games at the Staples Center in Los Angeles during August 2003 was a showcase for young men and women performing daring stunts on their skate-boards, skates, and bikes. While practice and more practice reduces the risk of injury, the risk-takers provide a steady supply of patients for emergency rooms and physicians.

The conflict between safety and pride also plays itself out in team activities. Football, as played in the United States, is a good example. Young boys playing in city leagues are taught to "suck it up" when they get bruised and banged around in practice and in games. Winning becomes a dominant theme, and the players who hit the hardest, run the fastest, and play with the most abandon get the top kudos from their coaches and appreciative parents. Everything is done to develop team spirit and to instill the desire to push oneself to one's limit for the sake of the team. Thus a player is not only "Johnny Jones," but "Johnny Jones, Viking." With this team identity, one risks injury not only to raise one's own status, but to raise the status of the team.

ENDURING PAIN FOR IDENTITY

Team image and team pride can become even more intense when individuals and their teams get to represent their schools and then their nations. Then we can talk about school pride and national pride. These can be extremely strong incentives to risk injury and push oneself to one's limits and beyond. An example is the two-day 130-mile race held in Japan known as the Hakone Ekiden, which keeps millions of Japanese glued to their television sets and fifteen ten-member all-male squads from Japan's universities trying to win for the glory of their schools and national pride.

The race is extremely grueling, with one stage of the race course going up a mountain where runners sometimes battle snow and ice, heavy winds, and freezing rain. If one member of the ten-member team has to drop out then the whole team is disqualified, which brings dishonor to that member. As one runner remarked in a telephone interview after being disqualified, "I was so sad, had so may regrets, and was in shock because I'd done something from which I could never redeem myself." He told the interviewer that he even considered suicide. The runners, imbued with an overwhelming need to bring honor to their schools and be worthy of their national identity are willing to endure fatigue, dehydration, pain, injury, and any other obstacle that gets in their way. As an eighty-year-old former runner remarked in a television documentary, "The true pleasure is found after going through agony. There's no play without struggle and agony."[6]

While the genetic programming to protect and preserve life and physical well-being evolved early in evolution and is well entrenched in human beings, protecting and preserving our sense of self and identity is also very well entrenched by now, even though, like us, it was a latecomer in evolution. And the interaction between these two evolutionary programs is not only played out in children, but continues to be played out in adults, families and social organizations. In many circumstances, a challenge to one has come to be used as a test of the other. For example, in the rites of passage to adulthood of many societies, youngsters must endure physical pain, suffering, and even mutilation. Enduring the pain in the ritual means that their identity with their group or social organization is solidified, and they are accepted by the other members. In essence, the initiate must choose between the protection and preservation of his or her physical well-being and the preservation and enhancement of his or her sense of self or identity. The group pressure to endure acts a strong incentive to tolerate ritualized physical punishment such as lying motionless on the ground while being bitten by hordes of ants,[7] having a tooth pounded out,[8] or being sexually mutilated.[9] Undergoing such a ritual is like taking a loyalty oath.

In modern western cultures, presenting an individual with a stark choice between physical suffering and the preservation or enhancement of identity through group acceptance has been limited to specific groups such as fraternities, sororities, and some cult groups. However, the ordeals individuals have to go through to become police officers, soldiers, and football players contain sizable elements of this conflict. Street gangs make extensive use of ritualized physical punishment to ensure that a newcomer is really motivated to take on the identity of the group. There are even slogans to push individuals toward accepting physical distress in order to enhance their physical image, their stamina, and their sense of worth. One such common slogan is, "no pain, no gain." And while cosmetic surgery uses anesthesia to reduce pain and suffering, people are willing to risk permanent disfigurement in order to improve their body image and sense of self. A recent phenomenon is the widespread acceptance of body piercing, anywhere and everywhere, in order to make an identity statement. The bottom line is that the conflict between one's physical well-being and one's sense of self has been around as long as modern humans, some 200 thousand years or more.[10] The universality of the conflict and the ways in which it manifests itself in different cultures strongly suggests that it fits the ideas of Dr. Carl Jung's archetypes and collective unconscious.[11]

IDENTITY WRAPPED AROUND A CAUSE

The conflict between life and self-worth or between safety and pride takes on a new dimension when self-worth and identity get wrapped around ideological causes, patriotism, religious fervor, and a sense of retributive justice. Under these circumstances, individuals may feel a calling which spurs them on or a group identity that subsumes their entire existence along with the realization that the group supports their acts. Thus they become driven and willing to risk life and limb.

For example, take the the story of Julia "Butterfly" Hill, the daughter of a preacher from Arkansas, who felt a calling to protect California redwood trees from being cut down for timber by Pacific Lumber Company. She found a way to climb up a 200 foot-redwood tree, destined to be cut down, and set up a "home" among its branches on December 10, 1997. She had to ride out winter storms eighteen stories above the ground with only a tarpaulin to protect her, and she had to be ready for accidents caused by other trees being cut around her. Many environmental groups supported her efforts and helped her out with water and food. She gained worldwide attention for her actions and became the world's most famous tree-sitter. She finally came down on December 18, 1999, after Pacific Lumber agreed to save the tree in which she had made a home. That was 738 days after she went up. She continued her protective efforts after she came down by founding the Circle of Life Foundation.[12] Just how many people are motivated enough to endure two years at the top of a 200-foot redwood tree?

Then there is Shahram Hashemi, who, on September 11, 2001, was on his way to the Bank of New York on Wall Street, where he worked as an intern, when the second plane crashed into the south tower of the World Trade Center. He first helped some women get into the lobby of the Bank of New York who were covered with dust and frozen with shock. He then went back to the World Trade Center to help out, despite the smoke-filled air and the raging fire. He was given a protective fire jacket by one of the firemen and joined a team of other individuals who became a volunteer fire brigade. Later he was given the task of bringing buckets of water to slake the thirst of firemen at Ground Zero. In the end, he too had to be rescued by a mobile triage unit when he became trapped in the rubble of a collapsed forty-seven-story building, and was evacuated to a hospital on Staten Island. A few days later he saw a picture of himself on the back page of Newsweek, wearing the fireman's coat and with a respirator hanging around his neck but, unlike other firefighters in the photo, without a helmet. When others recognized who he was he was interviewed by the press and asked what had motivated him to go back to Ground Zero to help out. He replied, "That is what Islam taught me to do, to help others, to sacrifice my life in order to bring peace. I could not have forgiven myself if I had walked away."[13]

Dogged persistence in the face of adversity and danger seems to characterize individuals who are motivated by causes to protect others, promote equality and fair treatment, and push for greater freedom. They frequently end up bumping heads with governments and authorities who are resistant to their causes. Protecting and preserving life and physical well-being applies to groups, organizations, and nations as well as to individuals. A vivid example of an individual willing to risk her safety for a cause that totally consumes her identity and that strikes fear into the government is that of Daw Aung San Suu Kyi.

Myanmar (formerly Burma), the country of Suu Kyi's birth, became an independent nation in 1948, a year after Suu Kyi's father was assassinated while fighting for Burma's independence. She was two years old at the time of her father's death. When her mother was appointed ambassador to India in 1960, they moved to New Delhi, the capital of India. Suu Kyi was fifteen years old at the time. While in India she was exposed to Mahatma Gandhi's philosophy of nonviolent resistance. She attended Delhi University and then enrolled at Oxford University in England. She met her future husband in England, married in 1972 and raised two sons.

In 1988 a movement toward democracy gained momentum in Burma, and Suu Kyi was drawn into the movement. In August of 1988 she addresses a rally in Rangoon, the capital of Burma, and remarked, "I could not, as my father's daughter, remain indifferent to all that was going on. This national crisis could, in fact, be called the second struggle for independence." However, in September a military coup took over the government, and gatherings of more than four persons were banned. An opposition group called the National League for Democracy (NLD) was formed, and Suu Kyi became its secretary-general.

Suu Kyi defied the ban imposed by the military regime and vowed, after the death of her mother in December of 1988, to serve the people of Burma "without fear of the personal cost." Thus, she set out on a long road of challenging Myanmar's military rulers and advocating nonviolent protests to obtain freedom for the people of Burma. She was threatened, intimidated, and placed under house arrest for "endangering the state," and she was only allowed visits from her immediate family. She went on a hunger strike, which incited protests by the Burmese public. The regime offered to free her if she would leave Burma, but she refused until the country was returned to civilian government and all political prisoners were freed.

In 1990 Myanmar's military rulers allowed general elections and Suu Kyi's party, the NLD, won 82 percent of the parliamentary seats contested. But, the regime ignored the vote, refused to allow the parliament to convene, and jailed the NLD's elected candidates. Suu Kyi was detained and denied visits even from her immediate family, and all outside contact was forbidden. Her plight came to the attention of the world, and governments around the world urged the Myanmar government to accept the election results. The secretary-general of the United Nations called for Suu Kyi's release. After being awarded prizes for human rights in 1990, she was awarded the Nobel Peace Prize in October of 1991 "for her nonviolent struggle for democracy and human rights." The award was presented in Oslo, Norway, on December 10, but since she was still in detention, Suu Kyi's sons accept the award. From her detention she announced that she would use the $1.3 million prize money to establish a health and education trust for the Burmese people. In the same month, her book, *Freedom from Fear* was published.

Sui Kyi, in May 2003, made her strongest statement against the regime . She said, "The NDL must stand up firmly to achieve the results of the elections of 1990. To ignore the results of the 1990 elections is to have total disrespect for the people and is also an insult to the people." In July 2003 a group of Asian and European foreign ministers called on the government of Myanmar to release Sui Kyi and other NDL members from prison.[14]

In September 2003 Suu Kyi was hospitalized for major surgery and discharged toward the end of the month to her home, where she again was placed under house arrest. Nothing seemed to have changed.[15] For the last fifteen years Sue Kyi has pushed for the democratization of Myanmar and endured intimidation, imprisonment, physical and personal attacks, and restrictions on travel and who was allowed to visit her. All this because of her convictions, which made up her sense of self and her identity. It seems as though she is willing to suffer endlessly if she has to in defense of her cause, in which her identity is totally immersed.

MARTYRS FOR A CAUSE

The founders and prophets of worldwide religious movements are examples of people who have been willing to stand up for their beliefs and convictions in the face of ridicule, persecution, and even death. There is Muhammad for Islam, Jesus for Christianity, and Moses for Judaism. A nineteenth-century martyr, Joseph Mukasa, who was the first Ugandan missionary among the group of missionaries known as the Martyrs of Uganda to be executed, succinctly presented the martyr's state of mind, "A Christian who gives his life for God is not afraid to die." [16] Certainly "Moslem" or "Jew" could easily be substituted for "Christian."

The next step forward in pitting one's life against one's identity that is wrapped up in a cause, is to deliberately kill oneself in the belief it will significantly further the cause. Here, for example, is a description of an action taken by a university professor who was trying to attract the world's attention to the mistreatment of women in Iran.

> In a crowded public square in Tehran, a woman removes her government-mandated facial scarf and and ankle-length coat. By baring her face, she is breaking Iranian law. Shouting "Death to Tyranny! Long Live Freedom!" the woman pours gasoline over her body and sets herself ablaze.

The woman was Dr. Homa Darabi, an internationally known feminist and the first Iranian ever to be accepted into the American Board of Psychiatry and Neurology. Her sister, Parvin Darabi, coauthored a book about Dr. Darabi called *Rage Against the Veil*, which was presented at the Center for Inquiry West on April 25, 1999.[17] Confirming the validity of this cause, the 2003 Nobel Peace Prize was given to Shirin Ebadi, an Iranian jurist who has fought for women's equality in Iran for many, many years and whose clashes with conservative clerics landed her in jail in 2000.[18]

The use of suicide to further a cause seems to have been taken to a new level by Palestinian suicide bombers in Israel, whose intention is to take as many Israelis with them as possible. The United States recently referred to them as "homicide bombers," but the newspapers continue to refer to them as suicide bombers whenever an attack occurs. The number of young Palestinians willing to kill themselves in order to kill Israelis seems to grow larger with each bombing incident. This is a phenomenon that has gained worldwide attention and appears to have made the intentional taking of one's life an almost everyday affair.

PROFOUND MEDICAL ISSUES

The clash between life and identity can become a very somber and fateful human drama when one is faced with a terminal illness that impairs one physically and produces constant pain or deprives one of activities that have been cherished and sustaining parts of one's life. My mother, for instance, put up with nine years of cancer treatment, including three operations, and came to the realization that there was no cure and that she could only look forward to more and more suffering until the cancer killed her. I was with her during the last moments of her life, when she decided she had had enough. She stopped eating, withdrew into her childhood once again, and started talking to her father, who had been dead for at least thirty-five years. I was informed by her doctor the next day that my mother had died. While it was heartbreaking for me to watch someone I loved struggle with this conflict and finally make a decision to end her life, it is a decision I have to respect. I still ask myself if there was something more I could have done to make her want to live. But in the end, the choice was hers. Sometimes there is no choice when death comes, and the conflict between death with dignity and prolonged suffering does not have to be faced. But when it has to be faced it is a heart-rendering decision.

A retired couple married for fifty-five years, apparently faced such a choice. The husband had Lou Gehrig's disease, according to the newspaper, and his wife had Alzheimer's disease. Both were in a residential treatment home living in the same small apartment complex, but due to her wandering and his poor physical condition they were told that they would have to be separated. One day they both signed out of the facility, went back to their former home, and committed suicide. They left a note stating they "wanted to be together forever." According to family members, this was not an impulsive decision, as they had talked with their family about the situation and their plan to leave this world together. Their daughter considered their actions as their last act of dignity[19]

Most religions, if not all, adhere to the principle that only God has the power and wisdom to determine matters of life and death. "It was God's will," is a commonly heard assertion regarding events of unexpected tragic consequence. Throughout theological teaching there resides the belief in predetermination. Expressions that encompasses this belief include, "I guess it wasn't my time to go," "if God wants you there's nothing you can do about it," and "God keeps a journal on everyone." When advances in the treatment of depression are added to religious beliefs, there seems little or no reason for anyone to feel he or she has has a legitimate right to consider ending his or her own life.

If someone succeeds in ending his own life, religion must assume that he acted inappropriately in that he tried to play God, and the mental health establishment may feel that it has failed the individual, in that treatment for depression was not successful. Neither religion nor the mental health profession leaves much room for suicide as a legitimate act, even though an individual chooses to give up his or her life in order to preserve a sense of self or identity that includes dignity, self-respect, and self-worth. The fact that many people are willing to risk or even give up their lives in order to sustain or elevate their image, reputation, self-worth or dignity shows how powerful this built-in component is in human affairs. This is one very important message of the psychological immune system.

Proponents of the view that a person has the right to determine when he wants to end his own life frequently clash with the opponents of this view in state legislatures over the issue of doctor-assisted suicide. In the United States, doctor-assisted suicide is legal only in the state of Oregon. In the rest of the world, only Switzerland, the Netherlands and Belgium allow this practice. Aside from religious opposition, opponents of doctor-assisted suicide fear that depressed individuals, who could be helped will become victims, and that once the door is open, judgments about which cases are legitimate and which are not will be subjected to family, social, financial, and political pressures. Thus far, the opposition has spoken with a more forceful voice than the proponents.

A recent study using neuroimaging has backed up the significance of the "sense of self" as a real entity. When individuals are psychologically injured by social exclusion felt as rejection, the pain registers in the same area of the brain as physical pain.[20] This suggests a possible physical foundation of our conscious self, and that evolution has made it a priority to protect, preserve, and enhance our sense of self and identity, as proposed in the psychological immune system.

Thus, while medicine can be seen as an outgrowth of our effort to protect, preserve, and/or enhance our life and physical well-being, the mental health profession can be seen as an outgrowth of our effort to protect, preserve, and/or enhance our sense of self and identity. Both physical and mental health practitioners need to be aware that conflicts between these two components of the psychological immune system often develop when their clients have issues concerning their physical well-being and their sense of self at the same time. Medical evaluation and treatment stir up questions of one's ability to get through an illness, one's judgment regarding how long one waited before seeking medical help, and whether or not one has been singled out by the unknown forces of the universe. Such questions make us take stock of our toughness, resilience, and adequacy; all part of our sense of self. Mental health evaluation and treatment stir up questions regarding genetic predisposition, brain functioning, and past stress on the body; all part of our physical well-being. Thus, it is important for physicians to anticipate the stirring up of a patient's anxiety about his or her sense-of-adequacy during treatment and for mental health practitioners to anticipate the stirring up of a patient's anxiety about an underlying physical condition causing his or her emotional problems.

ADDING PROPERTY AND POSSESSIONS TO THE EQUATION

One of the basic tenets of the psychological immune system is that we are genetically programmed to protect, preserve, and/or enhance our property and possessions. This includes real property, intellectual property, and items that we call our own. Property and possessions can be protected with the same intensity that life and identity are protected.

So what happens when we add the weight of property and possessions to that of life and physical well-being and weigh the combination against sense of self and identity? Or, what happens when we add the value of property and possessions to that of our sense of self and identity and weigh the combination against the value of our life and physical well-being? And how does the protection, preservation, and enhancement of property and possessions stack up against life and physical well-being combined with our sense of self and identity?

To better visualize the different combinations, they can be put down in an abbreviated form as follows:

Let LF/WB = life and physical well-being; Let PT/PS = property and possessions; and let SOS/IDT = sense of self and identity.

The first combination which weighs life and property against sense of self, could be written as (LF/WB + PT/PS) vs SOS/IDT.

The second combination which pits life against property and sense of self, could be written as LF/WB vs (PT/PS + SOS/IDT).

The third combination which balances life and sense of self against property, could be written as (LF/WB + SOS/IDT) vs PT/PS

In essence, the first combination asks under what circumstances an individual would favor his sense of self and identity (pride, self-esteem and self-worth) over his life and physical well-being plus his property and possessions. The second combination asks under what circumstances an individual would choose his life and physical well-being over his property and possessions plus his sense of self and identity. The third combination poses the dilemma of an individual having the choice of risking his life and sense of self in order to protect and preserve his property and possessions.

Children at school are confronted with this last dilemma when they meet a bully who threatens to take their property or possessions and hurt them if they tell anyone. This happened to me on the way home from the Y, when two bigger kids wanted my money and it happened to my son in junior high school (middle school) when a bigger kid with a knife demanded his milk money. Probably every child has a story to tell about having to decide whether to give up a possession in the face of intimidation or stand his ground and risk being physically attacked. Make no mistake, these conflicts spotlighted by the psychological immune system are universal and continue to confront humans all over the world. They are not easy to deal with and require a flexible approach. For instance, my son decided that if he didn't have any milk money in his pocket then the bigger kid would leave him alone. So, he hid his money in his shoe and after several confrontations with the bully with no money in his pocket, sure enough the bully stopped bothering him. It was not the way I wanted to handle it, but I had to respect my son's desire to solve the problem by himself. While he didn't raise his self-esteem by standing up to the bully, he was able to take pride in the knowledge that he had outsmarted the bully, saved his milk money, and not gotten hurt.

Would you stand up to somebody with a weapon who wanted to hijack your car? Would you confront a person who was robbing your house? I confronted such a person when I was a graduate student. I was sleeping on the couch trying to catch a few winks before studying again for my finals. I heard rustling noises, opened my eyes and there was a man going through my wallet that I had left on a table. Using a technique I had learned in my criminology class, I shouted at him "get the hell out of my house," and he complied by running out the screen door. It did boost my self-esteem since it turned out so well, but my heart was racing with greyhound-speed and I was very happy there was no physical confrontation. My dog "Buddy" whom I depended upon to bark at any intruder was sound asleep. After the robber ran out of the house, I yelled, "Buddy, Buddy wake up!" Buddy lifted his head up, let out one bark, and went right back to sleep. Had Buddy barked before, he would have saved me from making an agonizing choice of what to do.

The second combination, which pits one's life and physical well-being against one's property and possessions plus one's sense of self and identity, was dramatically highlighted when Saddam Hussein was captured in Iraq. He chose to protect and preserve his life and physical well-being at the expense of his property and possessions and his sense of self. Many of his countrymen called him a "coward" for making this choice. They thought he should have put up a fight to preserve his pride and possessions at the expense of his life and physical well-being. He did not take the route of the patriot or the martyr.

The colonists who came America in the seventeenth and eighteenth centuries were constantly faced with the combination of conflicts listed above. The British searched homes and shops for contraband with no warrant, British troops were quartered in people's homes without the owner's consent, and both land and possessions were seized with inadequate or no compensation. The British enforced laws with little regard for "due process" and treated the colonists arrogantly.[21] Thus, individuals were faced with choosing their life and physical well-being at the expense of their property and possessions as well as their pride and self-esteem. Those who chose to protect their property, possessions, and pride had to pay with their physical well-being and even their lives.

Thus, the British were the bullies, and the framers of the U.S. Constitution were very aware that governments could act in an arbitrary and overbearing way if not checked by the rules and laws of the country. The first ten amendments to the Constitution, which make up the Bill of Rights, were designed to protect people from the arbitrary power of the government that could take away their lives, their property, their liberty, and their good names. These are things, I believe, that people try to protect, preserve and enhance. The First Amendment gives people the right of free speech, freedom of religion, a free press, the right to peaceful assembly, and the right to petition the government to redress grievances. These are rights that enhance people's sense of self and provide them with a way of taking on the government. The Third Amendment affirms the sanctity of the home, while the Fourth Amendment protects citizens against unreasonable search and seizure of their persons, papers and effects. The Fifth Amendment prohibits the government from depriving individuals of their life, liberty, or property without due process of law and gives citizens the right to refuse to testify against themselves. Justice William Brennen, Jr., stated that searches with nonspecific warrants were "the single immediate cause of the American Revolution." [22]

The third combination listed above asks whether there are situations in which a person is willing to put his life and identity on the line in order to protect, preserve, and/or enhance his property and possessions. A person's willingness to do so would probably depend upon his sense of the magnitude of the threat against him, the person's evaluation of his chance of success in defending his property and possessions, and the value the person places on his property and possessions. That person would most likely have to have the attitude, "Just try and take my property or my possessions and see what happens to you!"or "You can take my property or possessions over my dead body." More often, though, what one hears is that property or possessions can be replaced, but not life so don't try to to be a hero.

Property and possessions can, however, have symbolic significance in addition to their monetary worth. They can represent status, personal worth, and the sweat and tears spent in acquiring them. Intellectual property can represent the talent and creativity of its authors, be it a painting, photograph, song, poem, or story. Furthermore, property and possessions can be used to protect one's life and physical well-being-for example a home, a car, a hideaway, a gun, or a bullet-proof vest. Thus, the conflict outlined above-property and possessions vs life and identity- is not always clearly defined . This certainly complicates the conflict, because an individual may not be aware of all of the ramifications that property and possessions have for him or her. Money certainly falls into this category.

Because property and possessions are so relevant to any social structure, people are hired to protect property and possessions at the risk of their lives and sense of self. This certainly characterizes police and firemen, who are continuously called upon to protect and preserve both public and private property and possessions. The risk to their lives and physical well-being as well as their sense of self and identity is inherent in their jobs, which they understand before they take the jobs.

If they don't do their jobs well they can be subjected to both public ridicule and self- condemnation. So, in order to tackle the conflict between property and life plus sense of self, society has seen fit to compensate the individuals well who take on the risks involved. They are given both status and power as well as a good wage.

CARING FOR OURSELVES VERSUS CARING FOR OTHERS

This last issue brings up the other principles of the psychological immune system and how they enter into the conflicts that have been explored so far. These are the principles that apply to those individuals we love, care about and/or identify with. While police and firemen are hired to protect and preserve the lives and property of citizens they may not know, family members are programmed to protect, preserve and/or enhance the lives, property and sense of self of other family members. They also extend this protective program to groups they care about and identify with. This can take the form of "proud to be a member of," "this group is like my family," "I feel like I really belong here," and "I love my country." Threats to family members or groups one identifies with are acted upon just as threats to oneself. An outside observer would say that an individual who defends family and cared-about groups is showing loyalty to them.

Protection, preservation, and/or enhancement of oneself can conflict with that of others one loves, cares about or identifies with. For example, a teenage mother who was walking through the Arizona desert for four days in 110-degree heat had to decide whether to drink the water she had and save herself or give the water to her eighteen-month-old daughter. When the border patrol found them, only a few ounces of water remained in the toddler's bottle. The mother was found dead of dehydration.[23] In another instance a ten-year-old boy fell through the ice in a twelve-foot deep pond. His older brother, who was nineteen, dived in after his younger brother to try and save him. Unfortunately, both died.[24] Both stories exemplify the conflict between the protection of one's own life or well-being versus the life or well-being of others and show how life events set up this type of conflict. The resolution can go either way and can be a "spur-of-the-moment" decision.

Other conflicts can arise between one's sense of self and the sense of self of other family members or between one's sense of self and the life or well-being of family members. In many Middle Eastern countries, for example, daughters dating without their fathers' permission-even daughters in their twenties-is considered an act of dishonor to the father and family. This can incite acts of violence against the daughter by the father or other family members. This type of conflict could be labeled as the sense of self and identity of the father and family vs the life and well- being of the daughter. To abbreviate, let SOS/IDT(S) = sense of self and identity of oneself (in this case, the father and family); and let LF/WB (O>lv) = life and physical well-being of others one loves or cares about (in this case, the daughter). Then the conflict becomes : SOS/IDT (S) vs LF/WB (Olv).

A conflict of this type ended tragically for the twenty-four-year-old daughter of a Jordanian family when the father discovered that his daughter had dated a man behind his back. He stabbed her to death to restore the family's honor. This type of killing is known as "honor killing" and, according to the U.N. Population Fund, happens to at least 5,000 women each year. It takes place in the countries of Pakistan, Afghanistan, Yemen, Lebanon, Egypt, and Jordan among others.[25] Even a twenty-nine year old woman is not exempt from dishonoring the family name by marrying someone she loves instead of someone chosen by her father. As a living example, a twenty-nine-year old woman stated in a lengthy interview that her father, who was a wealthy landlord and powerful provincial politician in Pakistan, had vowed to kill her for refusing to marry her cousin, as had been arranged since they were children. She said that one of her brothers who came to take her back home had promised to "cut her to pieces." [26]

One may well ask how a daughter whose father loves her, can be the object of his desire to hurt or even kill her. The explanation based on the psychological immune system is that the father's honor and that of the family trumps the life and physical well-being of the daughter, and that this outlook is sanctioned by the culture in which the family resides. Thus a threat or direct insult to the father's or family's honor(their sense of self and identity) triggers a desire to retaliate against the source of the threat or insult, and when the desire to retaliate is sanctioned by the culture, this pushes the desire into action. This parallels how the biological immune system works when it detects a threat or physical "insult." It directs its protective arsenal of chemicals and cells to neutralize or eliminate the source of the threat. However, it doesn't require a sanction from the culture at large, as the psychological immune system may, to put its destructive forces to work.

Thus, people can act in desperate and seemingly despicable ways toward family members when they feel their sense of self or identity is threatened, especially if their identity is tied to a position of power or high status in an organization. This was the case in Russia when a powerful police official learned that his newly born granddaughter was afflicted with a disease of the joints and looked deformed. He saw his granddaughter as a lifelong stigma, and he feared that she would be a constant threat to his reputation and the family's good name. So, he arranged with the help of some doctors in the local hospital to have his granddaughter sent away to an orphanage and to tell the mother, his own daughter, that her baby had died. Years later, when the truth came out and the grandfather was asked why he did what he did, he stated, "But I had neighbors, and they had a freak and it was in a wheelchair and looked like a monster. And for thirty years they went past my window, and I thought, 'Why should my children suffer like this?'" While he was ill in a hospital his daughter brought him a picture of her child - his grandchild - when she was three years old. He threw the picture down on the bed and exclaimed, "What now? Shall we declare this to all the world? Shall we ruin ourselves? Why did I meddle in this business?" It was as though he were trying to convince himself and his daughter that he did what he did for her and not for himself. His daughter could not forgive him for what he did and, in the end, he lost both the trust and respect of his daughter.[27]

There are many other conflicts generated between the components of the psychological immune system that involve the protection or enhancement of things relating to oneself versus things relating to those one loves, cares about, or identifies with. These types of conflicts, which occur in every family, are enough to turn parents gray at an early age. They occur between siblings, between parents and their children, and between the parents themselves. They can be as trivial as trying to decide who should get the biggest portion. For example, I recall fighting with myself when dishing out T-bone steaks to the rest of the family. Should I really give in to my desire and take the biggest one, or let someone else have it? It was a small conflict over "mine versus theirs," with the outcome reflecting on me. This type of conflict also characterizes siblings fighting over their property and possessions, which can represent their sense of self and identity. If the property has great personal value, the conflict can become very intense. Parents can hear, "But they didn't ask me if they could use it or borrow it. I don't touch their stuff," or, "If they touch my stuff one more time I'm going to do some bodily harm."

What can parents do to prevent or ameliorate these conflicts between their children or between their children and their friends. First, parents have to know that prevention can be difficult. They can ask themselves what can they do to prevent conflicts between themselves and their mates or friends? This is not an easy question to answer. When these conflicts are played out in the world at large within and between social organizations or within and between nations, which happens daily, the same question can be asked, namely, how can these conflicts can be prevented? In the thousands of years that civilization has been in existence so far, no one has come up with an answer that everyone agrees with. So, we are left with the practical question of how these conflicts can be worked out to the satisfaction of the parties involved without having to resort to force and violence.

PRACTICAL APPLICATIONS

My use of abbreviations and notions in the form of an equation may help clarify how the use of the psychological immune system can help resolve some of the conflicts mentioned above. First, one has to remember that the psychological immune system is made up of six separate components; three relate to oneself, and three relate to the individuals and groups one loves, cares about or identifies with. The components can be labeled as follows: S:1, S:2, and S:3 are the three components relating to oneself; and O:1, O:2, and O:3 are the three components relating to the others. Now a variety of equations can be set up. We can have;

$$(S:1 + S:2 + S:3) \text{ vs. } (O:1 + O:2 + O:3),$$

$$\text{or } S:1 \text{ vs. } (S:2 + S:3) + (O:1 + O:2 + O:3).$$

In the first equation, the power or influence the components exert on the individual seem equal, while in the second equation the power or influence the components exert on the individual seem very unequal and favor the right side of the equation.

Thus, if five components are lined up against one component, the probability is that an individual will decide against the lone component and be more forcefully swayed by the other five. This inequality, if used constructively, can be the basis for resolving many conflicts that arise. For example, as a parent or a teacher you have certain expectations about the daily activities your children or class will follow. They are expected to go to school and attend class unless ill or injured. They are expected to do homework when assigned. The children are expected to take responsibility for the orderliness of their room or desk. They are expected to follow the rules, such as waiting their turn if others are present and not pushing, shoving, or being obnoxious. They should know where trash goes and what to do if their shoes are muddy.

Inevitably, there comes a time when a child does not do what is expected of him or her. When asked to live up to your expectations, he or she says, "I don't feel like it," or " That's a stupid rule, and I don't have to follow stupid rules," or "No, I'm not going to do that homework, period, and I'm not cleaning up my room or straightening out my desk." The child may even draw a line in the sand and say, "I don't have to listen to you, you can't boss me around anymore." As one preadolescent put it, "I don't wanna, I don't hafta, and I ain't gonna."

According to the principles of the psychological immune system, this conflict can be expressed as the parent's or teacher's sense of self and identity versus the child's sense of self and identity.

Each has his own pride, sense of status, and a sense of what he or she will or won't put up with. Using abbreviations previously given, if SOS/IDT(S) stands for the parent's or teacher's sense of self/identity and SOS/IDT (C) stands for the child's sense of self/ identity then the conflict can be represented as follows: SOS/IDT (S) vs. SOS/IDT (C).

The parent's or teacher's sense of self and identity is challenged, which he or she can feel immediately. This produces the instant urge to use power and put the youngster "in his place." This can take the form of a physical threat, a threat to the child's freedom, a threat to the child's property or a threat to the relationship that the parent or teacher has established with the child. What may come out of the mouth of the parent or teacher goes something like this: " What do you mean you're not going to do your homework? What do you mean you don't feel like it? What do you mean you're not going to listen to me? Who do you think you're talking to ? Who do you think you are? That attitude will bring you nothing but trouble. You had better think twice about what you're saying." As the father in Bill Cosby's monologues would declare, "I brought you into this world, and I can take you out."

If you threaten your child's physical well-being then the above equation becomes SOS/IDT (S) + LF/WB (C) vs SOS/IDT (C), with LF/WB (C) standing for your child's life and physical well-being. In essence, your child now has to weigh his or her sense of self and identity (pride, self-worth), against his or her physical well-being and his or her concern about your sense of self and identity (which can come to their awareness via your reaction to their statements or your behavior in the form of anger, hurt, disappointment, disgust, etc.). If you add a threat such as taking away the child's allowance or freedom to ride his or her bike, skateboard, or scooter then you've added property and/or possessions to the equation. If PT/PS (C) represents your child's property and possessions, then the equation now becomes:

The SOS/IDT(S) + LF/WB (C) + PT/PS (C) vs. SOS/ID (C). Now your child has to weigh his or her sense of self and identity against his or her physical well-being, property and possessions and the concern, respect, or love for your sense of self and identity. You can make the left side of the equation even longer by threatening to take away the child's privilege to use any of your property or possessions, such as tools or makeup; to borrow money; or to use your cell phone or car. Thus, if PT/PS (S) stands for your property and possessions then the equation would look like this: SOS/IDT (S) + PT/PS (S) + LF/WB (C) + PT/PS (C) vs SOS/IDT (C)

Your child now has to weigh maintaining his or her sense of self and identity at the expense of his or her physical well-being, property and possessions, your property and possessions and your sense of self and identity. That's a heavy load to battle against. The only other component that can be added to the left side of the equation is your life and physical well-being. This would be represented by, LF/WB (S). To make your child aware of this component, you would have to say something to the effect, "You're killing me with your attitude," or,

"You're going to drive me to an early grave if you keep acting like you do," or " All this stress you're creating is going to send me to the hospital." Of course, if your child doesn't believe you, your statements will have little impact on your child. If your child does believe you, then this component will add considerable weight to the left side of the equation.

Thus far what we have are threats against the various components of your child's psychological immune system in order to counteract your child's decision to protect, preserve and/or enhance his or her sense of self and identity by rebelling against the expectations, rules, and obligations that you, as a representative of society, have imposed on your child. In your mind these expectations, rules, and obligations are reasonable, and will help your child adopt a more mature relationship with society. So you feel compelled to stand your ground and win the confrontation with your child by using whatever leverage you can.

Your child has challenged your authority and , like all people in power, you're going to fight fire with fire. I mean, try challenging a policemen, a judge, or the government and watch them use the same tactics against you and (unwittingly) against the components of your psychological immune system. Your life and physical well-being, your property and possessions, and your sense of self and identity will all be threatened eventually. In addition, the authorities may label you unpatriotic, un-American, and disloyal, which works on your identification with your community and country and makes you feel guilty for letting your community or country down. This is the same tactic parents use to make their children feel remorse or guilt for letting them down. How well this works depends on how attached you are to your community and country and how attached your child is to you. The greater the attachment the more sensitive one is to criticism from the community or the parents. This fits in well with the attachment theory that is so prevalent in psychology today and which has been championed by Dr. Daniel Siegel of UCLA, among others. [28]

While the practical benefits of understanding the psychological immune system can be seen when conflicts arise between individuals or between individuals and authority figures, thus far, we have examined only the use of threats. Threats often do help resolve conflicts, as any authority figure can attest, but they can also backfire, for they can leave resentment and revenge fantasies in their wake. This is because backing up threats relies on the use of force. Moreover, if tolerance of physical and emotional pain are criteria for evaluating oneself, then threats become a motivation to test oneself by resisting rather than conforming.

Now, if the left side of the equation we've been constructing contained items that were positively pulling on the child's psychological immune system and were seen as motivating the child to give up his stance against your rules and standards, it would make your job considerably easier and prevent resentment and the desire to get even. The goal, therefore, is to replace the threatening components with ones that act positively on the child's psychological immune system and encourage a desire to go *toward* these items, rather than *away* from threats.

Here's a little example that happened when my granddaughter and two of her friends, all between four and five years of age, were about to go to my granddaughter's house for a play date. I was going to transport the three children, myself, and my wife in our van which has three rows of two captain's chairs each. The front and middle row chairs have lap and shoulder belts, while the last row of chairs has only lap belts. We had two booster seats that were designed for the lap and shoulder belts and one child's car seat that had its own belt restraints. One of the booster seats belonged to my granddaughter, Sarah, and one belonged to her girlfriend, Taylor. The other girlfriend, Lulu, was to sit with the child's car seat in the last row with my wife sitting beside her. Everything was all set up, and we ushered the three playmates into the van for a day of fun with each other. Sarah got into her booster seat and Taylor got into hers, which was next to Sarah's.

My wife said, " Lulu, why don't you get into the back seat, and I'll sit right next to you, okay? " Lulu shook her head "no" and said something to the effect that she didn't want to sit in the back. "But my wife will be sitting right beside you, Lulu, and it's a short ride to Sarah's house," I said. Tears welled up in Lulu's eyes, and she insisted that she would not ride in the back seat. She said she wanted to sit next to Taylor or Sarah. So I asked Taylor if she minded riding in the back seat, and she replied that she did mind. Next I asked Sarah if she would do me a favor and ride in the back seat and let Lulu sit in her seat. Sarah did not want to give up her seat, thank you, and so there we were in the situation where Lulu didn't want to go along with the plan and the other two friends were of no help either. I next asked the girls if anybody had a plan to fix the situation we were in. Sarah mentioned something about trading seats along the way, but this didn't seem to help because nobody wanted to sit in the back seat to get started.

The situation boiled down to what we, the adults, wanted versus, what they, the children wanted. This fits into the equation already mentioned, namely: SOS/IDT(S) vs. SOS/IDT(C) where SOS/IDT(S) stands for the sense of self and identity of ourselves (me and my wife) and SOS/IDT(C) refers to the sense of self and identity of the children (the three girls). As adults, authority figures, and heads of state, we didn't have to stand for the resistance to our plans and the lack of cooperation we encountered. We could have pulled rank and made demands backed up by threats to their freedom, their plans to play with each other, or their physical ability to stop us from carrying out our plans. If we include threats to their freedom of movement and their inability to stop us from physically depositing one of them in the back seat as part of their physical well-being, we can include this in the left side of the equation. And if we threatened to deprive them of the books and toys they would be able to play with, then this would be a threat to the property and possessions they would have access to. With these additions, the equation would look like this:

SOS/IDT (S) + LF/WB (C) + PT/PS (S) vs SOS/IDT (C) where LF/WB (C) stands for the life and physical well-being of the three girls and PT/PS (S) denotes our property and possessions they would have access to.

These threats represent a potentially automatic reaction to being challenged and the common attitude that we adults are in charge, not the children, and we don't have to put up with their nonsense and tendency to act "childish." And my guess is that we could have accomplished our plan of putting someone in the back seat if we had instituted these threats. However, this had the potential of getting the play date off on the wrong foot, creating hurt feelings followed by anger, and possibly ending the play date early with someone crying, "I want to go home." Instead, the object became to replace the threats to the components of the psychological immune system with things that would *enhance* the kids' psychological immune systems and help overcome their resistance, represented by SOS/IDT (C) on the right side of the equation. This follows from our desire to protect, preserve and enhance the sense of self of our granddaughter and her friends.

For example, we could have been told the girls that the back seat has special powers and anyone sitting there would get stronger, taller, or prettier. Or that the back seat would make their backs stronger and straighter, and they would be healthier. Or that if they made a wish in the back seat it would have a good chance of coming true. If they believed any of this, it could have acted as a positive incentive and a challenge to their resistance. That would have addressed the life and physical well-being component of their psychological immune system.

The other component that could have been addressed is property and possessions. Instead of threatening to deprive them of property and possessions, we could have offered them some incentives such as toys, ice cream, or stickers . I know already that many parents and teachers would consider this "bribery" and would object strenuously to rewarding negative behavior. The belief is that the children would learn that by acting negatively they could get what they wanted. In a sense, then, the argument becomes that by offering a reward the children would get two rewards, namely: the "bribe" and the satisfaction of getting their way against adults. This argument leaves little room for negotiation and compromise, and sends a strong message that when you're in charge and have the power you can do what you want. This power differential is often felt by workers in large corporations and can lead to resentment. An example is the recent workers strike against Krogers, Vons, and Albertsons. Of course, when a child takes a position against the adults in charge that could put the child in physical danger or at risk of losing a valued object, then a definite stand has to be taken. But most circumstances do not rise to this level of peril.

Although it is difficult and sometimes aggravating, it behooves us, if we love our children, to allow them to come out of a situation without a sense of loss to their worth, status, or self-esteem. If adults always get their way by using threats, intimidation, and power, then children, in order to feel a sense of worth or esteem, will have to wait until they also get power and status and are able to use intimidation themselves. Bullies and gangs rely heavily on intimidation to gain status.

In the case of the three girls who refused to sit in the back seat, I took two of the components of the psychological immune system and attempted to make them exert a positive pull so that resistance would be given up willingly rather than in order to avoid the threats. I utilized the relationship I had with my granddaughter, which is covered in the psychological immune system by her love, concern, and care for my sense of self and identity and which is abbreviated as SOS/IDT (O>lv). I also made use of the property/possession part of her immune system by offering to have a book she liked read to her and stickers for being a good sport. This component is abbreviated as PT/PS (C). In essence, what I said was that if she sat in the back seat, her grandmother would read her a book of her choice, that we had on hand, while we were traveling, she could get stickers and I would appreciate it very, very much. So, these three components and her awareness that I cared about her pulled against her resistance and she was willing to comply. At last, everybody was pleased. Sarah also got kudos from my wife. So the play date started off on a positive note and the rest of the day went very well. In essence, I had looked after Sarah's sense of self and identity, and she had shown recognition of mine.

The final equation representing the positive components competing with her resistance, (where SOS/IDT(O>lv)[1] =

Sarah's concern for my sense of self and identity, PT/PS(O>lv)= My property and possessions that she will have access to, PT/PS(C) = The property and possession offered to Sarah, and SOS/IDT(O>lv)^2 = My concern for Sarah's sense of self and identity of which she is aware), is as follows:

$$SOS/IDT(O>lv)_1 + PT/PS(O>lv) + PT/PS \ (C) + SOS/IDT(O>lv)_2 \ vs \ SOS/IDT(C)$$

This example points out that, as parents and teachers, we would be wise to look for incentives and enhancements to replace the usual threats that we use to solve the conflicts that arise between children and between ourselves and our children if we're going to train or teach our children to handle conflicts in the future. If compromise and negotiation are neglected in favor of threats, power and force then that's what we can expect our children to carry into their future. When we look around the world we can only hope that compromise and negotiation are favored as a way of resolving conflicts. Substituting incentives and enhancements in place of threats is not an easy exercise but my guess is that the more we practice the better we would become. The principles of the psychological immune system, expressed in equation form, offer a way to visualize how combinations of threats and incentives can be used to motivate and induce changes in behavior. While the example focused on children the same format can be applied to adult interactions and behavior.

In summary, the psychological immune system provides a model for understanding what internal and external forces affect our behavior and the behavior of others. This model can suggest strategies for handling the inevitable conflicts that arise within ourselves and between ourselves and others. It is a system that tells us how our inbred nature to protect, preserve, and/or enhance our life, our property, and our identity direct us when we come up against our environment, our social structures, and our experiences. It also lets us know that many, if not all, of our social structures and national priorities are manifestations of the psychological immune system.

This last conclusion will be explored further in the coming chapters.

CHAPTER VI

Applications to Groups, Organizations, Nations and Societies
A New Perspective on the Past and Present

OUR SYMBOLIC BRAIN

When my granddaughter, Sarah, was eighteen-months-old and sitting at her little wooden table with a pencil and paper, she started drawing small lines on the paper. As she drew the individual lines she declared, "This is Mommy, this is Daddy, this is Bro-Bro (her brother), and this is Nanna (her grandmother)."

This caught my interest, and I asked her to tell me about her lines again. She repeated what she had said before and was very definite about which line stood for which family member. It is intriguing that at such an early age children become aware of representing things in the real world with just a scratch mark. This symbolic ability may not be very startling to an adult because it is commonplace for children that age and older to use marks, drawings, Play-Doh, and dolls to represent things in the world around them. While it is a commonplace ability, it took evolution millions of years - at least 6 million - to get animals to show this skill. We are those animals with this remarkable endowment.

If we jump to age five, children can draw a circle and have the circle stand for or represent a seed, an apple, a tree, a person, a city, a state, a nation, the earth, our solar system, a galaxy, or the universe. They can also talk about some of the qualities of the object represented by the circle. Again, this is not a spectacular feat for a child this age or older. And the older, more experienced, and more knowledgeable children become, the more they can add to and elaborate on the qualities of the objects represented by verbal and nonverbal symbols. While most of us fall far short of creating such an elaborate and profound symbolic formula like Einstein's $E=mc^2$ which represents the relationship between energy and mass, or Watson and Crick's double-helix configuration that portrays the structure of DNA, we nevertheless use the same processes of conceptualization and symbolization.

VISUALIZING SINGLE ENTITIES

Even relatively young children can understand the concept of "family" and provide the names of the individuals who make up the family. They can grasp the idea of the family getting larger when new children are added or the family getting smaller when older members die. It is generally accepted that families have a history and that members can recite the saga of the family:

the hardships that were faced, the good and bad times that were experienced, and the resolve and sense of purpose that helped them stay the course. With sufficient information an outsider looking in could rate the family's health and well-being, its status in the community, the value of its property and possessions, and could provide a fairly accurate appraisal of how proud or ashamed members were to be part of the family. In essence, the life and well-being, the property and possessions, and the sense of self and identity of the family as a whole can be recognized, written about, and reliably agreed upon. That's why historians can write about the Rockefeller family, the Kennedy family, the Sinatra family, and the Bush family. That's the reason social scientists can dwell on family stability, structure, relationships, and family interaction. It also explains why the family can be the focus of counseling and therapy. Like the individual, the family can be treated as a real entity, with life, property and an identity. These are the components that the psychological immune systems of family members are programmed to protect, preserve, and/or enhance.

Like the family, cities can also be thought of as having a life and physical existence, accumulating property and possessions, and having an identity. One of the Los Angeles supervisors, for example, talked about Los Angeles, known as the City of Angels, regaining its "image and identity" by sponsoring a professional football team once again. Many cities have a recognized image and identity, such as Philadelphia, which is called The City of Brotherly Love; New York, which carries the title of The Big Apple; and San

Francisco known as the Golden Gate City. In Europe, some well known cities with images and identities are Paris, referred to as The City of Love; Nuremberg, called the Gingerbread City; and Budapest, known as the Pearl of the Danube.

Cities, like individuals and families, have existence. They occupy a given space, they can grow or shrink, and they can die. The State of California is home to many deceased cities and towns. For example, the town of Eldoradoville in Los Angeles County was a mining community that was washed away by a flood in the early 1900s. It was never rebuilt, and the only remains are several abandoned mines in the area.[1] Zurich, a town in Inyo County, named by the residents because of the jagged peaks of the White Mountains, "died when the rails were pulled up from Tonopah, Nevada to Keeler, California."[2]

The State of Arizona has had a host of cities and towns that have experienced an untimely death. For example, Canyon Diablo in Coconino County sprang up in 1880 when railroad construction was halted until a bridge could be built over the canyon. It became a lawless town in which saloons, gambling houses and brothels ran twenty-four hours a day. After ten years the railroad bridge was built over the canyon, and this caused the demise of Canyon Diablo.[3] A town in Arizona, near death, goes by the name of Greaterville, located in Pima County. It came to life around 1879 when men came looking for gold, and about 500 residents, mostly Mexicans, made a living packing in and selling very scarce water. Its post office was closed in 1946 after the mining activity dwindled. Supposedly, there are still a few residents living in the city.[4]

A corporation is another entity that can be thought of as having a birth, a life or existence over time, accumulating property and possessions, developing an image and identity, and eventually dying if not nourished properly. As a matter of fact, in 1886 the U.S. Supreme Court, in the landmark case of Santa Clara County v. Southern Pacific Railroad, determined that corporations could be defined as "persons" and were protected by the Bill of Rights, including the First and Fourteenth Amendments.[5] This ruling still holds today, and corporations have expressed their First Amendment rights through their cash contributions to individuals running for congress and the presidency. The old saying "money talks" has been extended to include "and the talk is protected by the First Amendment."

Certainly, many corporations have grown considerably since the 1886 Court decision, and by 1997 fifty-one of the world's hundred largest economies were corporations, not countries.[6] Corporations have an existence, but can also cease to exist, dissolve, or die. They can lose their property, possessions, and financial holdings. They can lose their reputations, images, and status in the economic market and in the eye of the public. Recall the savings and loan debacle in the late 1980s and early 1990s, when Lincoln Savings and Loan went under and Silverado Savings and Loan Association soon followed. Congress, for the first time in U.S. history, agreed to bail out an entire industry as opposed to a single corporation.[7] The thrift crisis cost $153 billion, with the U.S. taxpayer shelling out $124 billion and the thrift industry giving $29 billion.[8] In 2004 we saw the failure of Enron, Global

Crossing, WorldCom Inc., and TWA. In April 2004, PG&E ended its three years under U.S. bankruptcy court protection.

In a corporation, since the shareholders elect a board of directors and the board elects officers-usually a CEO, vice president, treasurer, and secretary-who are supposed to follow the policies of the board and manage the day-to-day activities of the corporation, the individuals involved make the corporation part of their own identities and have stakes in the assets of the company. The corporation becomes, as it were, an extension of the psychological immune system of the individuals involved. Therefore, Managers are naturally alerted to safety and survival issues, the acquisition and protection of property, and transactions that affect the image and identity of the corporation. However, it behooves them to be aware of whether their decisions stem from their own self-interest or from the best interests of the organizations they represent. This may be a perpetual conflict that has to be faced day in and day out. Dr. Herbert Simon, a Nobel prize-winning economist and noted psychologist, outlines the above problem as follows:

> Individuals also strive rationally to advance their own personal goals, which may not be wholly concordant with the organizational goals, and often even run counter to them. Moreover, individuals and groups in organizations often strive for power to realize their own goals and and their own views of what the organization

should be. To understand organizations, we must include all of these forms and objectives of rationality in our picture. We must include human selfishness and struggles for power[9]

The above discussion applies as well to other organizations besides corporations. The behavior of religious and civic organizations, for example, can also be seen as an extension of the psychological immune systems of the individuals involved in running them. Like individuals, these organizations protect, preserve, and/or enhance their lives and physical well-being, their property and possessions, as well as their sense of self and identity. Covering up mishaps, mistakes, and the harmful actions of its members-like the Catholic Church's coverup of its priests molesting children-can become part of the protective stance of organizational behavior when fear of losing security, wealth, or image comes into play.

As organizations become larger and larger, the interaction between their members can become more complicated and groups represented by the organizations or groups of people with whom the organizations interact can become more diverse. Thus, an organization, as a single entity, is subjected to various demands and pressures from the groups and individuals under its umbrella. This statement applies equally well to nations, which may contain varied ethnic groups, different religious groups, multitudes of workers belonging to different occupations, and political groups representing diverse schools of thought. However, nations, like families, corporations, and other organizations, are systems put together and run by people. Therefore, a nation can also be conceptualized as a specific entity with a birth, a life, and an existence. A nation also has property, possessions, an image, a sense of itself, and an identity.

Historical data provide accounts of how nations came into being, but there are also mythological narratives about their beginnings. A story about Japan goes that the female god Izanami and the male god Izanagi stood on the floating bridge of heaven and stirred the ocean with a jeweled spear until it curdled. This created the first Japanese island, Onokoro. Izanami then gave birth to the eight islands of Japan, but when she gave birth to the god of fire, she was badly burned and died.[10] Another story centers on the origin of Australia. According to the native people, the country came about "when the ancestor beings, ancient humans and animals, sang the land into life. The ancestors walked along the land and sang the mountains, hills, gullies, rivers, plants and all the other natural phenomena into reality."[11]

So it appears that our ancestors were able to conceptualize nations as single entities with beginnings, just as we still do today. Furthermore, nations, kingdoms, and empires can cease to exist or die just as individuals, families, corporations and cities. Tripolitania, as an example, became an independent country in 1711 after being part of the Ottoman empire for more than 150 years. As one of the North African Barbary Coast states, it plundered shipping in the Mediterranean, which led to the

Tripolitan War with the United States in 1801. It came under Turkish rule in 1835, and then under Italian rule in 1912. During World War II its territory was the scene of fierce fighting between British and German forces, and in 1951 it and two other provinces were combined to form the independent Kingdom of Libya. The provinces were dissolved in 1963, and the country of Libya remained.[12]

The Ottoman empire, mentioned above, is another instance of a living aggregate of nations and territories that, after many centuries of conquest and power, lost its life and physical well-being. It all began in the fifteenth Century when the Ottomans, under Muhammad II("the Conquerer"), destroyed the Byzantine empire and captured its capital, Constantinople, in 1453. Under Selim (1467-1520) and his son Suleyman I("the Magnificent"), the Ottoman empire became the largest in the world. The Ottoman sultans also held the title of caliph, the spiritual head of Islam. Ottoman power began to decline in the late sixteenth century with the destruction of the imperial fleet, and in 1699 the empire had to relinquish Hungary. With the Russo-Turkish wars and wars with Austria and Poland, the empire came to be known as the "sick man of Europe." It lost most of its remaining territory in the Balkan Wars of 1912-1913, and sided with Germany during World War I. Thereafter, postwar treaties dissolved the empire. [13]

So nations and even empires have characteristics that are the same as those of families, corporations, and cities, namely: they have a life or existence, property and possessions, and an identity. Like individuals, they protect, preserve, and/or enhance these attributes because they are governed by individuals and individuals make up their membership. Using this prospective they can be said to have psychological immune systems and can be understood via the principles and operations of their psychological immune systems. This means they are vigilant for threats against their existence, property or identity and alert to opportunities to enhance their lives, wealth, or images. It also means they are prepared to take action, and do so, when they feel their lives or physical well-being, their property and possessions, or their sense of self and identity are threatened. They also take action when they feel these same components can be enhanced by opportunities they are aware of. Furthermore, conflicts develop between the components of their psychological immune system, just as in individuals, and they struggle mightily to resolve them.

RESPONSES TO THREATS AND OPPORTUNITIES

FAMILIES

Just as the the cell is the basic unit of the body, the family is the basic unit of a society or nation. Therefore, there is an interactive effect. What happens in a society affects the family, and what happens in the family affects the society. Threats to and opportunities for families can come from without via the economic and social conditions they are faced with, or they can come from within by way of the stability, instability, accomplishments, and behavioral difficulties of its members. It is up to the family leaders, usually the parent or parents, to provide stability and direction to the family. They provide role models for the children to follow and are extremely important as anchors or safe harbors in times of danger. A lost parent in a mall or playground can produce panic in young children just as a lost child can produce panic in a parent. These characteristics and features are right out of our primate past and have survival value for the family.

The glue that holds the family together is the love, caring and concern for each other. These emotional bonds are nowadays referred to as "attachments" by mental health practitioners and researchers, and are considered to be programmed into our brains. As theoretical models and research data indicate, there can be "secure" attachments and "insecure" attachments, which carry their own influence on the future behavior of family members.[14] Secure attachments make children more receptive to parental standards because children are sensitive to and do not want to incur parental indifference or rejection, whereas insecure attachments produce less receptivity to parental standards.[15] Therefore, some believe that insecurely attached youngsters are more prone to join gangs and be more open to antisocial behavior.

While love, care and attachment seem to be important elements in most families, Meg Taylor, Ambassador from Papua New Guinea to the United States from 1989 to 1994, points to obligation as an important element in the families of New Guinea. She writes,[16]

The most powerful thread is the family, the clan. The manner in which we care for one another, protect one another, and are loyal to one another appears in the way we carry out our obligations to one another. The duty of obligation takes many customary forms: in trading relationships, in the exchange of pigs, in a bridewealth, at funeral rites. The common thread here lies in the honoring of relationships between families and clans that enables harmony to prevail. The continuity of such customs from one generation to the next honors our past, gives us our sense of values, and contributes to our feeling of belonging.

When economic conditions deteriorate, jobs and money are hard to come by and families suffer. The stability of millions of families was threatened during the two major economic depressions of 1893 and 1929. According to the book _A People's History of the United States, 1492-Present_, the 1893 depression saw 642 banks go under and 16,000 businesses close their doors. In the 1929 depression, more than 5,000 banks failed and about fifteen million people were put out of work. The heads of families were desperate, and many took desperate measures to ensure the well-being of their families.

For example, in the Great Depression of 1929, veterans of World War I went to Washington to demand that Congress pay off their government bonus certificates early so that they would have money to live on and care for their families. More than 20,000 camped across the Potomac River from the capital on a piece of land known as Anacostia Flats. They built makeshift shelters of cardboard, packing crates, tarpaper roofing, and anything else they could find. When the bill to pay off the bonus certificates passed the House but was defeated in the Senate, most of the veterans and their families refused to leave. President Hoover ordered the army to evict them. General Douglas MacArthur was put in charge of the operation, with Major Dwight Eisenhower as his aide and George S. Patton as one the officers. The army, using tear gas and setting fire to the makeshift shelters, eventually forced the veterans and their families to leave, but not before two veterans had been shot to death, thousands had been injured by the gas, and an eight-year-old boy was partially blinded.[17] When families decide to fight for their existence, it takes considerable force to thwart their efforts.

During the Depression, families throughout the United States lost their homes. They stayed at public shelters, slept in public toilets and under bridges, and built shantytowns along railroad tracks. Many waited in food lines run by nonprofit organizations or the government, and some even scavenged in garbage cans.[18] Some families organized to help themselves and sold things on the black market. Crime went up substantially, and so did suicides. As stated before, families who are desperate do desperate things to maintain their lives and well-being. But watching other family members suffer, on top of the loss of property, status, and self-reliance, can be so devastating to some that they lose their desire to continue life's struggle.

ORGANIZATIONS

Competitors, whether in teams, organizations, or national enterprises, usually try to outdo each other in order to be at the top of the competitive pile instead of the bottom.

So it was with Kroger, Safeway, and Albertsons, which vied for customers in their desire to make the most profit, until a strike was called by the United Food and Commercial Workers union in November 2003. Suddenly they were all faced with the same threat to their profit and viability: customers who supported the strike and refused to cross the picket lines. Since customers are the lifeblood of these food giants, what did they do? They made a mutual-aid pact to share the pain of the labor strike in case the United Food and Commercial Workers union applied pressure unevenly. In fact, the union did. Pickets were removed from Ralph's stores, owned by Kroger, and concentrated on the stores owned by Safeway-Vons and Pavillions-and Albertson's. This resulted in the Ralph's chain setting aside $116 million to compensate Safeway and Albertson's for their loss during the strike. This was so unusual that California Attorney General, Bill Lockyer alleged that the pact violated federal antitrust laws. The food giants contend that the pact was a legal, labor-related exemption from the antitrust laws. As of this writing, the courts have yet to resolve this matter.[19]

In addition to union strikes, taxes are also considered a threat to corporate profit and hence to corporate stability. So what have corporations done about taxes? A General Accounting Office report showed that 61 percent of U.S. corporations paid no federal income taxes from 1996 through 2000. Of those that did pay income tax for the year 2000, 94 percent reported tax liabilities of less than 5 percent of their total income instead of the established rate of 35 percent. In addition, the percentage of federal income tax supplied by corporations has fallen from a high of almost 40 percent in 1943 to a low of about 7 percent in 1993. Eugene Steurele, a former Reagan administration tax official, explained the results as due to corporations moving their income to low tax-rate countries where they get the biggest tax advantage. Thus, companies have become more tax-savvy because their attorneys and accountants have become better at finding tax loopholes and tax reduction plans.[20]

In order to stay alive, some corporations, like Enron and WorldCom, have used the tactic of overstating their profits and understating their losses. It seems as though the pressure to keep a good thing going, when the CEOs and other managers had gained a substantial windfall, caused them to use tactics that were either questionable or downright illegal. While many CEOs don't cave in to this pressure, it is always there. Corporations have also resorted to strike-busting tactics, payoffs to officials, the use of illegal aliens in sweatshops, and a host of other maneuvers to protect, preserve, and enhance their lives and well-being-which to their executives is synonymous with profits. Of course, corporations also use legal and innovative strategies to stay alive by taking advantage of research, outreach, advertising and the ability to get help from the government when necessary. As an example, Chrysler Corporation was nearly bankrupt in 1979 when it hired Lee Iacocca as their president. In 1980 he persuaded Congress to loan Chrysler $1.5 billion, and he shifted the company's emphasis to more fuel-efficient cars. He also embarked on an aggressive advertising campaign. Within a few years, Chrysler was showing record profits.[21]

If CEOs, presidents, and executives of organizations are going to take credit for keeping their organizations alive and functioning, they must also take responsibility for sick and dying organizations. The excuse, "I wasn't aware that such-and-such was going on," is a pretty poor one, since these high-priced officials are hired to be aware of things that affect the survival and profitability of their organizations. This fits with the principles of the psychological immune system, which declare that individuals are acutely aware of situations that pose a threat to the life, property, or identity of themselves or the individuals and groups they are bonded to or identify with. It certainly applies to corporate directors whose job it is to maintain the viability of their corporations. If they identify with the corporation, that awareness is built into their psychological makeup. Claiming ignorance is like trying to ignore the elephant in the living room or turning a blind eye to the emperor who has no clothes.

NATIONS AND SOCIETIES

Considerable resources, wealth and energy go into the security and protection of a nation or a society because of its built-in predilection to stay alive and protect its physical well-being. This is the first principle of the psychological immune system. So we see, among a vast array of possibilities, the creation and maintenance of defense departments and armed forces, the development of education systems and spy networks, the establishment of economic programs and regulations, the funding and support of medical systems and research, and the formation of agencies and networks to protect national borders.

Like the biological immune system, which is programmed to keep out unwelcome intruders and and keep the body safe, the psychological immune system also directs government leaders to keep out unwelcome intruders so that a nation or society will be safe. They must identify unwanted persons and maintain a system to keep individuals out or detain them if they come in. However, nations and societies must guard against becoming overzealous and overreacting which even the biological immune system can do.

For example, Australia has a policy of detaining all applicants for political asylum who arrive without proper identification. They can remain in custody for years before the government decides their fate. Prime Minister John Howard maintains that he must take a strong stand against unwanted refugees because Australia, which has 19 million people, cannot absorb large numbers of refugees. With hundreds of children and their families placed in detention centers, a sense of hopelessness sets in. The refugees fear returning to the countries they came from and their requests for asylum are often rejected, so they are in a state of limbo. Some have gone on hunger strikes to protest their continued detention, and others have even attempted suicide. As one of the refugees stated, "People overseas still believe like we used to that Australia is a real humanitarian country. They will not understand until they are here, and then it is too late."[22]

The protection of society from unwanted intruders arises from the same fear that a society can become contaminated by physically and mentally handicapped people. This has caused some countries to institute eugenics programs to eliminate or sterilize such individuals before they can produce offspring to swell the ranks of the handicapped. Such a program was practiced in Japan from 1949 to 1996, during which time thousands of people were sterilized. A doctor's recommendation was required, along with the approval of a committee appointed by the government. Japan's Eugenics Protection Law was written in 1948 to "avoid the birth of defective offspring" which was supposed to include a broad range of mental and physical handicaps, hereditary diseases, and leprosy or Hansen's Disease.[23]

Japan is not the only country to institute eugenics programs in an attempt to keep genetically "inferior" people from contaminating the rest of society. For example, between 1907 and 1939 the United States sterilized more than 30,000 people in twenty- nine states, many of whom were in prisons or institutions for the mentally ill. Between 1935 and 1976 Sweden sterilized 60,000 people who were deemed genetically inferior. But the leader of all nations in forced sterilization was, of course,

Hitler's Germany. The vision of creating an "Aryan master race," led to the Law for the Prevention of Progeny with Hereditary Diseases in July 1933. Persons included in the program were the mentally ill, the retarded, the physically deformed, epileptics, the blind, the deaf, and severe alcoholics. It has been estimated that between 300,000 and 400,000 people were victims of the law. This was the forerunner of the systematic killing of the mentally ill and handicapped, which was started in about 1939. Many in the medical and psychiatric community supported Hitler's program.[24]

As well as being fearful of letting in unsavory immigrants and contaminating the society with genetic defects, nations also become suspicious, if not paranoid, of their own citizens during times of crisis. Executive Order 9066, issued by President Franklin D. Roosevelt following the attack on Pearl Harbor by Japan, reflected this paranoia. The order allowed the U.S. Army to round up more than 100,000 persons of Japanese ancestry living on the West Coast, most of whom were U.S. citizens or legal resident aliens, and relocate them to remote camps surrounded by barbed wire and armed guards. After the war, the Commission on Wartime Relocation and Internment of Civilians felt that the government's actions reflected wartime "hysteria." The public was mostly unaware of these internment's until the war ended. An article by Yale Law Professor Eugene V. Restow in *Harper's Magazine* in September 1945, the month the war ended, called removal of the Japanese "our worst wartime mistake." In 1988 Congress acknowledged that "a grave injustice was done." [25, 26]

WORKING ON CONFLICTS

As pointed out in Chapter V, individuals are most sensitized to threatening and opportunistic aspects of situations they encounter in regard to their life, property, and sense of self, as well as others they are close to. When such situations call for choices to be made among the six components of the psychological immune system conflicts develop, and these conflicts can become quite distressing. The same holds true for families, organizations, nations, and societies.

LIFE AND PHYSICAL WELL-BEING VERSUS SENSE OF SELF AND IDENTITY

(LF/WB VS. SOS/IDT)

For individuals, the conflict between one's physical well-being and one's sense of self, which was covered in Chapter V, starts at an early age, with most individuals willing to risk some physical injury in order to bolster their sense of self. This does not require much conscious contemplation, as the urge to avoid hurt and the urge to bolster one's sense of self come from the basic makeup of human beings. It takes special circumstances or situations within the social structure to bring out these opposing urges. How these urges manifest themselves in families, organizations, nations, and societies can get quite complex and convoluted, but behind the smoke, mirrors and complexity, the basic conflict remains.

FAMILIES

This conflict can develop when circumstances place a family in such a position that its action or inaction has profound consequences for its well-being and sense of self. This occurred, for example, during the Second World War, when Jewish families in Poland, Denmark, Holland, France and elsewhere were running for their lives from the Nazis. Other families, seeing their plight had to decide whether to get involved or look the other way. Some non-Jewish families got involved by turning in their fleeing countrymen to Nazi authorities. Other families known as "Righteous Gentiles" took in fleeing Jews and hid them. These families put themselves in grave danger. If the Nazis discovered what they were doing, they would face the same fate as the Jews-arrest, torture and concentration camps. According to the Yad Vashem Authority in Israel, about 20,000 Righteous Gentiles have been recorded in more than thirty-five countries.[27] However, most families chose not to risk their lives at the expense of injury to their sense of self.

Jehovah Witnesses were also hunted by the Nazis, and by 1939 an estimated 6,000 Witnesses were detained in prison camps. Many were tortured by the police in an attempt to make them sign a declaration renouncing their faith. However, when faced with choosing between their physical well-being and their identity, very few renounced their faith. All told, about 10,000 Witnesses were imprisoned in concentration camps.[28] It takes a strong conviction in a cause, a goal, a belief or a value system for any family to risk its life when circumstances ask them to make a choice. After all, fear of death or injury is basic to human life and is programmed into our brains. To override this fear requires emotions that take priority over fear of death or injury. Fear registers in the amygdala, an older part of the brain, while pride and identity most likely register in the neocortex, a newer part of the brain. Thus, the conflict can be conceptualized as the amygdala and the neocortex fighting for dominance.

Of course, it is possible that sometimes families or group leaders don't realize how great the risks are until it's too late and they are faced with the inevitable and they can't back down without losing face or appearing weak. The more people are watching or involved, the greater the pressure to stay the course in the face of danger. However, in great social causes where families band together, they are usually well aware of the dangers they face. This was the case in the civil rights marches led by the Rev. Martin Luther King and others.

The march from Selma to Montgomery, Alabama, in 1965 was an example of families willing to put themselves in harm's way to obtain civil rights that white citizens already had. It was a march that made people feel proud and more powerful than they had been before. The march started on Sunday, March 7, and resulted in attacks by police and state troopers, who fired tear gas into the crowd and severely beat the marchers. As one of the protesters recalled, "They even came up in the yard of the church, hittin' on folk. Ladies, men, babies, children -- they didn't give a damn who they were." After the death of a white minister from Boston named James Reeb, a federal judge ruled that the state could not block the march. When the march ended in Montgomery on March 26, 25,000 people had joined in a triumphant display of solidarity for the civil rights movement.[29]

The basic struggle to be and to be of some worth still faces many families today. The millions of families who find it hard to make ends meet have to resist the temptation to fudge on their taxes, gamble with the little money they have, work out some shady deals on the black market, and stay within the law. They are constantly faced with a conflict between their physical well-being and their sense of values. As one mother from the Congo, trying to raise four children on less than a dollar a day, stated after deciding to go into prostitution, "We're not bad people. This is how we have to live. This is how we put some food in our stomachs."[30]

The same struggle is made by families who confront issues that can tear the family apart, like divorce, adultery, incest, and interfamily abuse. Children caught in the middle of these problems try to hold on to both their physical well-being and their self-esteem which can be extremely difficult without outside support. For instance, children who are the victims of physical abuse try desperately to avoid further abuse by avoiding the abuser or avoiding the behavior they believe brought it on. They also try desperately to hold on to the belief that they are not as bad as their abusers would have them believe, or that the total fault is not theirs. So, their psychological immune systems go into overdrive, and they become super-aware of avenues of avoidance, escape, or protection and supersensitive to signs and signals when another abusive episode is near. At the same time, the abuser is also sensitive to signs of resistance or rebellion, and a cat and mouse game ensues. Unless the victims are unusually resourceful, they need help from the non-abusing parents, other family members, or social agencies in order to keep their physical well-being and their sense of self intact. Many families resist outside "interference," as they feel it is a blight on their family name and reputation. Their mantra is, "We can handle the problem ourselves." This does not leave victims in a favorable setting.

ORGANIZATIONS

While organizations are more impersonal than families, they also face the same conflict when their representatives do things that have the potential for damaging the very existence of the organizations. Then they must choose between owning up to the actions of their representatives, and facing the consequences or trying to cover them up . Although organizations can misjudge the consequences and make decisions based on misjudgments, the conflict that evolves nevertheless pits the physical well-being of the organizations against their sense of self or identity.

A case in point is the highly publicized sexual abuse scandals in the Catholic Church. The Church maintains an image and identity of a very moral, spiritual, caring, and socially responsible organization. The Church is also known for its vast financial resources, which can be considered the physical well-being of the church. Its priests are the backbone of the Church and carry both the physical well-being and the identity of the church on their shoulders. A tenet of the psychological immune system is that the physical well-being and the identity of organizations are both protected with the same degree of intensity, an intensity that has its roots in human evolution. This protection falls to the hierarchy of the church, namely the bishops and cardinals. The molestation of children by priests has the potential to damage both the image and physical well-being of the church. What have the bishops and cardinals done since the accusations came to their attention? They have tried to protect both the physical well-being and image of the Church by hiding the facts and trying to mollify the victims so they won't go public. The offending priests have been preached to, shifted to new parishes, and sent to counseling. An attempt has been made to handle the whole affair internally.

This scenario is not very different from that of families in which incest has occurred and the non-offending parent-usually the mother-has found out about it. Typically, she is in a state of denial because she foresees the devastating consequences to her family, especially if the husband is the breadwinner. Yet she feels that the moral standing and value system of the family has been violated. She usually confronts her husband and lets him know how terribly he has acted, and may even try to get him to promise, with his hand on the Bible, that he will never do this again. She tries to comfort the molested child by promising him or her that their daddy will never do this again. But, overall, she tries to play down the consequences of the molest and keep the whole affair in-house. She just wants the whole matter to go away like a bad dream. Many, many times the non-offending parent has to be pushed into acknowledging what has happened and made to see that her main job is to protect and help heal her child. The amount of shame, remorse, and guilt that emerges is an indication of the degree to which the values of the family have been violated. If the offending parent goes into therapy, the affair will come out into the open because the therapist, unlike an in-house Church counselor, is obligated by law to report the abuse. Thus the family conflict becomes very intense, and it usually takes outside pressure to bring things to a head.

So, in essence, the circumstances confronting the Church say "make a choice between your sense of self and your physical well-being." The Church's response is "I don't want to make a choice, and I'm not going to." And just like the situation in the family, when the affair comes out into the open, all hell breaks loose. The comments by A.W. Richard Sipe, a former priest turned psychotherapist who has counseled hundreds of priests with problems hanging on to their celibacy and who has done much research in the area of sexual abuse by Catholic clergy, brings these points home very candidly. He says of the Church hierarchy, "Some of them are so terrible. I mean, the plain lying that I've seen, bishop after bishop saying, 'No, this was never true, I don't know anything, I can't remember anything.' And sometimes the bishop just smiles. One bishop said, 'I only lie when I have to.'"

The Church's failure to choose the path of protecting its image and identity by confronting the sexual abuse openly and honestly and living up to their code of morality and sainthood, rather than protecting its physical well-being instead, has resulted in damage to both its physical well-being and its image. It has been estimated that the Catholic Church has paid out some $800 million in settlements already, although Mark Chopko, general counsel for the U.S. Conference of Catholic Bishops, puts the figure closer to $300 million. But, as everyone realizes, not all of the victims have come forward yet, so the final toll on the church's finances has still to be determined, And the image of the Catholic Church has been badly tainted by the scandal. As Cardinal Bernard Law, the senior member of the U.S. Roman Catholic hierarchy, said in his homily at the Cathedral of the Holy Cross in Boston, "We do not always make holy decisions." [32]

As of this writing there is a movement afoot to subpoena the personnel files of priests who are alleged to have molested minors since January 1, 1988, the cutoff date for criminal prosecution based on a Supreme Court ruling. However, many civil suits are still pending and Cardinal Roger M. Mahony's lawyers have argued that releasing Church records violates the legal privileges of the Church.[33] So it seems that because the Catholic church did not live up to its moral image, its physical well-being is being attacked from all sides. Many of the 195 dioceses in the United States are having a hard time staying afloat financially. The diocese of Portland, Oregon filed for bankruptcy in July 2004, and the Boston archdiocese recently settled 552 abuse cases for $85 million. St. Susanna is one of sixty-nine Boston area parishes scheduled to close by the end of 2004, but Boston Archbishop Sean Patrick O'Malley insists that the closings are unrelated to the financial problems caused by the sexual abuse scandals and settlements.[34] It appears the coverup is still going on, and the Church is still not ready to choose between its physical well-being and its identity.

On paper, many organizations have noble goals and express socially responsible values which, supposedly, make up a substantial part of their image and identity. When incidents arise which have the potential to threaten their financial standing or take a bite out of their profits, where the rubber meets the road, so to speak, then their image or identity is pitted against their physical well-being.

As an example, here are some identity statements made by some very large corporations.

#1. "Live our core values. Promote our corporate reputation. Make an impact in areas where business and societal need intersect through focused connected actions. Measure our performance and create an open dialogue with our global shareholders." (General Motors) [35]

#2. "We are a global family with a proud heritage passionately committed to providing personal mobility for people around the world. We are a leader in environmental responsibility. Our integrity is never compromised and we make a positive contribution to society." (Ford Motor Company)[36]

Needless to say, these companies have vast holdings, great wealth, and a strong determination to protect their lives and physical well-being, which translates into their profit. Let's look at some situations that have threatened these companies' profits and identities and see what choices the companies have made.

In 1965, Ralph Nader, an attorney and freelance writer, published *Unsafe at Any Speed: The Designed-in Dangers of the American Automobile.*[37] The book was a continuation of his research into the engineering design of automobiles, which he first made public in a 1959 article in The Nation entitled "The Safe Car You Can't Buy." The article declared, "It is clear Detroit today is designing automobiles for style, cost, performance and calculated obsolescence, but not-despite the 5,000,000 reported accidents, nearly 40,000 fatalities, 110,000 permanent disabilities and 1,500,000 injuries yearly-for safety."[38] One of the book's targets was the Chevrolet Corvair, a very successful compact rear-engine car from General Motors, which Nader faulted for a rear suspension system that could cause the car to skid violently and roll over.

So, now General Motors had a problem trying to decide whether it should favor its "core values" and its identity or try to protect its physical well-being by not losing any profit. What did it do? It decided to protect both by demeaning the source of the report, namely Nader. General Motors hired a private detective to gather information that could discredit Nader and even tried to set him up with hired women. A journalist, James Ridgeway, wrote about G.M.'s attempt to discredit Nader, which prompted Senator

Abraham Ribicoff's subcommittee on Executive Reorganization, that was investigating auto safety, to confront the president of General Motors, James Roche, and make him apologize.[39] The Corvair was discontinued in 1969.

In April 1974, the Center for Auto Safety, concerned with the safety of the 1971 Ford Pinto's fuel tank, petitioned the National Highway Traffic Safety Administration (NHTSA)-which came into being in 1970 after congressional hearings-to force Ford recall the Pinto. The petition was not acted upon. Then, in 1977, Mark Dowie, of Mother Jones magazine, published an article on the dangers of the fuel tank design, based on the documents by the Center for Auto Safety. He also cited internal Ford documents that indicated the company was aware of the fuel tank deficiency but had decided against any changes because of replacement or repair costs. Once again, faced with the conflict of stated values vs profit, the "Our integrity is never compromised" company chose profit. It took a jury's award of $125 million-later reduced to $3.5 million by the trial judge-to a passenger in a Pinto that had burst into flames after being hit by another car going twenty-eight miles per hour, and renewed tests by NHTSA, along with the publicity it generated, to convince Ford to recall all 1971 -1976 Pintos and have their gas tanks modified.[40]

A more recent example is the 1988 Consumer's Union report on Suzuki's Samurai sport-utlility vehicle, which claimed that the vehicle "easily rolls over in turns" and gave it a "not acceptable" rating. The report could have prompted Suzuki to re-evaluate the vehicle and make some changes. After all, Suzuki prides itself on being a company that has the public's interest at heart. But what did Suzuki do? It ignored the report and continued selling the Samurai until 1995. Then, in 1996, Suzuki sued Consumer's Union for $60 million, claiming that the "not acceptable" rating had caused sales to plunge and tarnished Suzuki's image. Suzuki apparently also tried to tarnish Consumer's Union's image by claiming C.U. had faked the tests on the Samurai. Suzuki sued again, and the case went to court in the year 2000 but the trial judge dismissed the lawsuit against Consumer's Union. Suzuki appealed the decision, and in the year 2003 the Ninth Circuit Court of Appeals sent the case back to trial. Before the anticipated trial could be held, an out-of-court settlement was reached.

Suzuki dropped their lawsuit and Consumer's Union clarified the statement "easily rolls over in turns," to mean in severe turns, not in routine driving conditions. All this despite one of Suzuki's own expert witnesses testifying that the company knew of 213 deaths and 8,200 injuries involving Samurai rollovers.[41, 42]

It seems that many companies don't realize that their images are tarnished not by others pointing out defective products, but by their own defense of their positions in order not to lose money- that is, choosing their financial physical well-being over their sense of self and proclaimed identity.

NATIONS AND SOCIETIES

Since nations and societies are rarely homogenous, they are forever evaluating their relationships with the various groups they comprise. How fairly, equitably, and humanely the groups are treated reflects the sense of self or identity of the nation or society. Oftentimes the slogan "the conscience of the nation" is used to convey its humanity and sense of fairness. How many nations would characterize themselves as treating their citizens unfairly or unjustly? My guess is, none! Yet when national resources, property, and wealth are at stake, the government of a country or the agencies that make up the government have to confront the same conflict that families and organizations do. What will they do when circumstances demand that they choose between their wealth and their sense of self, between their resources and their good name?

What did the United States do when Elouise Cobell, the treasurer of the Blackfoot Nation, asked for an accounting of unpaid money due the Indians for land leased to oil, mineral, timber and cattle companies? Land that the Dawes Act of 1887 allotted to indian families and individuals, and which the United States government held in trust because it didn't trust the Indians to handle their own real estate with the same level of competence that the Department of the Interior could. What did the government do? It chose to ignore her request in the hopes she would go away and stop bothering it so it wouldn't have to make a choice.

But Cobell was determined not to go away and enlisted a Washington, D.C., banking lawyer by the name of Dennis Gingold. Together, with the help of many charitable organizations, they raised enough money by 1996 to file a class-action lawsuit in federal court against the Interior and Treasury departments, on behalf of half a million Native Americans, for failing to fulfill their fiduciary duties to manage the trust.

The court, under judge Royce Lamberth, ordered the Department of the Interior, the Treasury Department, and the Bureau of Indian Affairs to produce records of the trust funds so that accountants could reconcile the balance and estimate of how much the Indians had been paid over the years. The government agencies could not produce the records as ordered, so the judge held the agency heads in contempt of court and imposed a fine of more than $600,000. Then, in December 1999, he issued a 126-page opinion against the government, calling the case "a shocking pattern of deception," adding "I have never seen more egregious conduct by the federal government."

The government appealed the case to the U.S. Court of Appeals, but to no avail. It was reluctant to push on to the U.S. Supreme Court. There was talk of the liability going as high as $40 billion, but no settlement seemed to be in the immediate future. As of 1999, a second phase of the trial to determine what the government owes had yet to be put on the court docket. The government had more than 100 lawyers assigned to the case.[43] At last, in May 2004, the United States Court of Appeals set a trial date with oral arguments to be held on September 15. Elouise Cobell, who was listed as the plaintiff, had this to say in a July 2004 memo to the 500,000 trust beneficiaries.[44]

> Unfortunately, the government has, so far, acted with
>
> the same bad faith in mediation that they have shown in

administering the trust and litigating the Cobell case. It is self-evident that to have any chance of success, mediation must have two participants who want to resolve the conflict. In this mediation, it has become obvious the government wants to resolve nothing.

What is a "fair and just resolution," you ask? A complete and accurate accounting of our trust assets-nothing more and nothing less. If the government wants us to give up our rights to that complete and accurate accounting, it must compensate each of the individual beneficiaries. It is that simple.

What the Cobell case brings out is that a national government, often to its own detriment, frequently places a higher priority on wealth than it does on its sense of fairness and justifies its actions by equating wealth with stability and self preservation. Yet when the government wants to define itself to its citizens and other nations, it places its sense of fairness before everything else. Does it always know what it is doing, or does it let fear run its policy? And is its fear a reflection of its vulnerability and feeling of fragility? If so, this leads to a hypersensitivity to threats and danger when little or none really exist, very much like the allergic reaction of the biological immune system.

How about a hypersensitivity to the danger of the Internet? The Internet opens up a world of ideas, interacting human beings, new cultures, new scientific discoveries, new and different values and ideologies, as well as a world of new products and where to find them. So one would think countries would be elated to have their citizens use computers to gain access to the Internet, right? Well, almost right! Let's take China, for instance. The Constitution of the People's Republic of China, adopted on December 4, 1982, states in Article 35, "Citizens of the People's Republic of China enjoy freedom of speech, of the press, of assembly, of association, of procession and of demonstration." Article 37 states, "The freedom of person of citizens of the People's Republic of China is inviolable. Unlawful deprivation or restriction of citizens' freedom or person by detention or other means is prohibited." Finally, Article 38 proclaims, "The personal dignity of citizens of the People's Republic of China is inviolable. Insult, libel, false charge or frame-up directed against citizens by any means is prohibited."[45]

With this constitution as its fundamental document, the People's Republic of China presents itself as a country that takes pride in upholding the rights and dignity of its citizens. So why should access to and use of the Internet be seen as some type of threat to the stability and well-being of the government? And even if the Internet is seen as a small threat, wouldn't an outsider predict that the government would place a higher priority on its sense of fairness and identity, based on the principles of the Constitution?

However, reports by Amnesty International, Human Rights Watch, the Berkman Center for Internet & Society, and Bobson Wong, a researcher with Internet Communications, all point to China favoring the left side of the equation when its physical well-being is challenged by its sense of fairness and identity. Wong, for example, notes that individuals have been arrested or detained since 2000 for (1) browsing reactionary websites that distort relevant facts and criticize the Communist Party; (2) publishing "subversive articles" on the internet; (3) spreading information on the banned Falun Gong spiritual movement over the internet; (4) criticizing government repression of the Falun Gong spiritual movement; (5) posting a letter on a web site from a mother of a young student killed during the Tiananmen Square demonstration; and (6) "incitement to subvert state power" because of ties to the online magazine Democracy and Freedom.[46]

China has resorted to blocking some Internet sites such as Amnesty International, Human Rights Watch, the Hong Kong Voice of Democracy and the Direct Democracy Center.[47] Amnesty International reports that there are more than forty-five million Chinese Internet users who could gain access to ideas and information censored in traditional media. Therefore, they maintain, China views the Internet as both "a boon to the country's rapidly developing economy," and "a danger to its own control."

To try to maintain control, China's Ministry of Public Security has tried sponsoring a large number of hackers to attack dissidents residing abroad. For instance, Tibetan independence groups report "an unrelenting barrage of e-mail viruses targeting their networks." Likewise, Falun Gong websites run from outside

China have been bombarded by hundreds of e-mail viruses daily. In May 2002 the entire site of a Falun Gong supporters' group was destroyed by a hacking incident.[48] Thus it seems that China's insecurity about the stability of its government leads it to over-react to minor or insignificant threats for fear they will turn into major and significant threats. As a result, China is willing to go against its own constitution.

This conflict in the psychological immune system between physical well-being and sense of self, which circumstances provoke, is not limited to the United States or China but touches every nation in the world. An issue that brings this conflict to the fore and with which countries around the world have been struggling since the Universal Declaration of Human Rights was ratified by the United Nations in 1948, is Torture.

Practically every county in the world has been willing to sign at least one document that proclaims the immorality and illegality of using torture, even of prisoners who have broken the law or been captured in wars. Since no one has forced any country to sign such a document, their doing so must mean that they accept this moral standard as their own and proclaim this standard as part and parcel of their self-image and identity. Yet when countries feel under threat, either from individuals or groups within the country or those outside the country, they seek to detain and arrest them. This is followed by interrogation and plans to neutralize or eliminate the individuals or groups. And more often than not, torture seems to be considered as an optionto extract information, obtain confessions, send an intimidating message to others, take revenge, or show the power of the state.

So now we have the conflict set up. Protecting, preserving, and/ or enhancing a country's physical integrity versus protecting, preserving, and/or enhancing the country's proclaimed international image and identity.

On December 10, 1948, the General Assembly of the United Nations adopted and proclaimed the Universal Declaration of Human Rights. The member states of the United Nations pledged themselves to live by this human rights document. Article 5 states, "No one shall be subjected to torture or to cruel, inhuman or degrading treatment or punishment."[49] This document still stands as a landmark in defining human rights, and it has been accepted by almost all member states of the United Nations.

In 1961, after the United Nations Commission on Human Rights requested a draft of "principles on freedom from arbitrary arrest and detention", The Declaration on Protection of All Persons from Being Subjected, to Torture and Other Cruel, Inhuman or Degrading Treatment or Punishment was adopted by the General Assembly in 1975, and a Covenant on Civil and Political Rights was ratified in 1976, becoming international law. This covenant forbids torture and inhumane or degrading treatment. Then a Code of Conduct for Law Enforcement Officials and a resolution entitled Principles of Medical Ethics were approved by 1982. These drafts, declarations, and principles ended in The Convention against Torture and Other Cruel or Degrading Treatment or

Punishment, which was adopted by the General Assembly in 1984 and became effective in June of 1987.[52, 53]

Thus, the 194 member nations of the U.N. have put a lot of effort into defining standards to be used with prisoners, captives, detainees, and those arrested for violations of national and civil codes of conduct. The standards adopted do not allow torture or degrading treatment. Almost all nations have signed one or more of the above named documents. In essence, their signatures signify their acceptance of those standard and tell the world that this is the image they intend to live by and that this image is incorporated into their sense of self and identity. Yet according to an analysis of human rights trends released by Amnesty International in June of 1999, "torture, 'disappearances' and extra judicial executions have escalated around the world in the past decade." The report covered 141 countries and said that 66 percent of the countries had used torture or ill-treatment. This means that at least ninety-three countries were still using torture.[52]

Since September 11, 2001 the "war on terrorism" has given countries extra incentive to favor "national security" over their stated international image or identity. A recent study, made during 2002, revised the number of countries still using torture to 106. Therefore, despite all the good intentions of making torture an illegal and immoral activity, it is still being used in the name of national security, as the August 2004 report by the U.S. Department of Defense on Abu Ghraib prison abuse so clearly demonstrates.[53]

In summary, the conflict between the two components of the psychological immune system, namely: life and physical well-being versus sense of self and identity, is triggered by events and circumstances that are sometimes unforeseen and other times anticipated. This conflict manifests itself in individuals, families, organizations, nations, and societies. Which side of the equation is favored and acted upon depends on the willingness of those concerned to put their life and physical well-being on the line for some principal, cause, belief, or doctrine that is the underpinning to their sense of self or identity. More often than not, life and physical well-being take priority over sense of self and identity. This is what allows corporations to favor profits over public concern and what allows nations to continue using torture.

As pointed out in Chapter V, there are a number of common conflicts that develop between the components of the psychological immune system because the social structure prompts individuals to choose between different priorities. Families, groups, organizations, and nations are also prompted, if not forced, to make choices because of the forces operating in national and international societies. Some of these conflicts are :

(1) life and physical well-being of oneself versus life and physical well-being of others (that one loves, is bonded to or identifies with).

(2) life and physical well-being of oneself versus property and possessions of others.

(3) life and physical well-being of oneself versus sense of self and identity of others.

(4) sense of self and identity of oneself versus sense of self and identity of others.

These conflicts include such issues as favoritism, fairness, and equality in families, organizations, and nations. They also allude to many provocative questions. How much of a risk will an organization or nation take to defend your life and possessions? How do societies determine what intellectual property and possessions can be copyrighted and privately owned, as opposed to being public property? How do families, organizations, and nations determine the worth of the human rights of their members as opposed to their own internal security? When do national values and national honor trump the values and honor of citizen groups?

Each of these questions deserves its own chapter, which is beyond the scope of this book. My goal is simply to point out that a psychological immune system exists which influences the issues individuals, families, organizations, and nations, struggle with and provides clarification to these issues. This helps shed light on the options that are available to deal with these issues. What will these issues be for the twenty-first century? This is the venture of the next and final chapter.

CHAPTER VII

The Relevance of the Psychological Immune System to the Twenty-First Century and Beyond

A Road Map for Life's Journey

CONSIDERATIONS ABOUT THE PSYCHOLOGICAL IMMUNE SYSTEM

We are in the twenty-first century with a psychological immune system that has come to us courtesy of evolution that alerts us to threats to and opportunities for ourselves and those individuals and groups we love, care about, and identify with. Once alerted, the system proceeds to protect us from threats and make use of opportunities in order to sustain us. This includes threats to and opportunities for our life and physical well-being (LF/WB), our property and possessions (PT/PS), and our sense of self and identity (SOS/IDT).

When we look around, we can see how the psychological immune system shows itself in our lives and in the cultures, societies, and nations that we have created and become part of. It has steered us to form kinship groups, develop protective strategies, create societies and cultures that provide avenues for the ownership of private property and the development of our sense of self and identity. Our predisposition to protect, preserve and/or enhance our LF/WB, PT/PS, and SOS/IDT is either activated or kept in check by the environmental and cultural forces we encounter in our day-to day-lives. It would be very helpful if we knew which environmental and cultural forces excite and which suppress the different components of the psychological immune system. It would also be grand if we could rely solely on the innate programs and responses of the system rather than having to learn new ones. Wouldn't our children like that!

If just sitting down and thinking brought sudden insight about the world and how it operated it would make things a lot easier. But, learning about the world we live in is a slow and tedious process, as any elementary school teacher can attest. It's a step-by-step, issue-by-issue, day-by-day procedure. If you've ever had the privilege of helping out in a preschool or kindergarten class, you would have noticed right away how many times the teacher has to repeat a lesson before the children get it right. Learning proceeds little by little, step by step, over and over again, until the errors become fewer and fewer and the responses become better and better. This formula applies not only to classroom learning but also to sports. Watch as coaches teach children soccer moves, football tactics, and the elements of basketball. In fact, practicing, practicing, practicing and learning by trial and error never stops, even in professional sports. More moves, more strategy, the continual elimination of errors and mistakes take on lives of their own as the games progress. How much and how often coaches grimace and yell are indicators of how effectively mistakes and errors are being eliminated. The goal in the classrooms and on the playing fields seems to be errorless performance-in other words, "perfection."

PERFECTION VERSUS ERROR

Recent studies have indicated that the human brain is programmed more toward the trial-and-error method of responding than the "ah-ha" or the sudden insightful response. For example, Joseph LeDoux's research indicates that the neural pathways from the brain's emotional center, the amygdala, to the thinking center, the frontal cortex, are much more prolific than the pathways from the cortex to the amygdala. He concludes from this that the job of the cortex is to prevent inappropriate responses rather than to produce appropriate ones.[1] In other words, the job of the effective brain is to catch and prevent impulsive but wrongheaded reactions to emotionally charged events. If bad reactions are weeded out, better ones are left. This certainly presents a good rationale for putting people who deal with emotionally charged events-like police, firemen, and medical emergency workers-through countless role-playing and practice sessions until they weed out faulty responses and replace them with correct ones. It makes good sense to use role- playing and rehearsal as tools to prevent unwise reactions in many different settings and under many different circumstances.

Furthermore, brain imaging studies of primates and humans have shown that the part of the brain that deals with intentional goal-directed behavior, the prefrontal cortex, responds more intensely and actively when monitoring negative performance than positive performance. This means it is more engaged when monitoring errors and mistakes than monitoring behavior that brings rewards. The research psychologists doing these studies conclude that the prefrontal cortex is extensively engaged in performance monitoring. This includes checking for failures and errors when seeking a goal, and helping the individual with performance adjustments like taking a more cautious approach or producing more controlled responses.[2] It seems our brain is programmed to deal with correcting mistakes.

How do errors and mistakes fit into the scheme of life? Considering that life on earth has continued for about 3.5 billion years[3] despite the many adverse conditions it has encountered, like extreme heat, cold, pressure, hurricanes, floods, fires, and volcanic eruptions, one would expect that mistakes and errors are not life's strong suit. Yet it is interesting to note that the most important process governing life's continuance, namely the replication of DNA chains before cell division, is not a flawless one. If anything should be perfect, one would expect that the process which passes on the code of life should be perfect or near perfect. But, if this were the case, new daughter cells that result from cell division would be exact replicas of their mother cells and change would be nonexistent. If there were no change over time, antibiotic drugs would encounter no resistant bacterial strains, and pesticides would not have to be continually changed to take care of agricultural pests. But, perfection is not the standard for the creation and passing on of life. Rather, diversity and flexibility characterize the scheme upon which life rests, and this comes from the flaws, errors, and mutations that accompany the replication of DNA and the differences that result. Once there is a continuum of differences or variability among offspring, natural selection can then choose those variants that can best adapt to a changing world.

The continuation of life, then, depends on the protective mechanisms that organisms develop to meet obstacles and threats to their existence. Changes in the environment lead to new dangers and offspring with the right protective mechanisms or those that have the flexibility to adapt to changes will survive. Our biological immune system encounters new and varied microorganisms every day of our lives and needs the flexibility to engage and destroy harmful pathogens before they get a foot in the door, so to speak, and destroy us. The medical and pharmaceutical industries have come about because of the inability of the biological immune system to take on and conquer all the pathogens that attack us or to take on and destroy errant cells that develop into cancer. The psychological immune system, in order to protect us, needs the same flexibility, for it encounters new and varied threats as societies change and bring new challenges.

Above, all, one has to remember that the psychological immune system is a protective system that has evolved from the basic thrust of life, and as such it is not perfect. It uses whatever resources are available to it and proceeds by trial and error and learning from its mistakes. In this sense, perfection then becomes the elimination of as many errors as possible, which is a never-ending process and relies heavily on our cortical activities. As a protective scheme, the psychological immune system relies on threat detection, memory, and learning from past mistakes, and it is a persistent built-in force that influences our motivation and behavior, which in turn influence our social systems and our governments.

PROTECT AGAINST WHAT

As in previous centuries, the desire to protect people we love is very much present in the twenty-first century because it is part of our genetic programming. We want to see our children grow, mature and become healthy and happy adults. While children want our protection, they also want the freedom to emulate what adults do so that they can feel a sense of accomplishment and add a notch to their sense of worth. An everyday event involving my granddaughter, Sarah, brings out these issues clearly.

When Sarah was three years old she wanted to cross the street by herself and tried to pull her hand away from mine. I held on and said, "You have to hold hands if you want to cross the street." She replied, "I can do it myself!" This remark prompted me to explain to her why doing so could be dangerous to her life and physical well-being. So I began, " A car could come down the street, hit you, and hurt you really badly. That would make me very, very sad, and I would cry and cry and cry."

My expectation was that she would grasp the danger of getting hit by a car and being hurt if she didn't cross the street safely and that I was protecting her from this danger because I loved her dearly. I figured she would say, "Okay Papa, I'll hold hands," and instinctively feel good because she was being loved. From the standpoint of the psychological immune system, I thought I was appealing to her built-in desire to protect her life and physical well-being and also give her sense of self and identity a boost. What I didn't count on was that my statement would be taken as an attack on her sense of self and identity and that it would arouse her desire to protect her and my sense of self and identity. So she had the task of convincing me that she was indeed competent to handle the situation but doing so without offending me-not an easy task for a three-year-old. But, she came back with this little gem: "It's okay Papa, I'll go into the house and get a band-aid and put it on my owie where the car hit me. So you don't have to cry."

In effect, Sarah was saying that she could protect her life and physical well-being if push comes to shove, and that I can could calm down and not be so concerned. In her mind, she was promoting her own competence and protecting me from feeling sad. While childish, magical thinking went into her answer, which severely underestimates the danger of being hit by a car, her thought processes can be understood as a reflection of the principle of the psychological immune system.

My granddaughter's statement reminded me of what I heard from a kindergarten class with which I was involved as a mental health consultant. When I asked the children what problems bothered them the most, they said, "Bigger kids picking on us, calling us names and hitting us." When I asked what they could do about this problem, I got a variety of answers. Aside from telling the teacher, principal, or their parents, they presented fanciful answers that reflected an exaggerated sense of power. Here are some of the solutions they proposed: "If they beat me up I'll just punch them right in the mouth." "I'll sock him in the nose." " I'll get my dad's dog to bite them." " Tell my dad, if I had a horse, to give me the horse and I would buck over them." "I'll run so fast they'll never catch me."

As we enter the twenty-first century we still have cars to contend with, older children picking on younger children, the magical thinking of children and the complexities of modern society, which always brings us new things to worry about. With its protective format, the psychological immune system impels us to be alert to dangers we face and to deal with injuries we receive whether they be physical or psychological in nature. If we cannot deal with given dangers and injuries or feel overwhelmed by them, we turn to the people we are close to, trust, and who we believe can help us.

Children are continually faced with dangers and injuries they cannot handle and generally turn to their parents first. If the parents are not available, they will turn to other family members-siblings and other relatives. If this doesn't work out, children will turn to peers and others they interact with. They will continue this process until they find someone or someway to deal with their dilemma, because the psychological immune system is programmed to handle threats in any way it can, making use of both innate or built-in responses and acquired or learned responses.

So one thing is certain: if the family is not available to handle threats and injuries children encounter, children will look elsewhere, even to their own fanciful ideas. This is true for threats and injuries to their physical well-being, their property and possessions, and their sense of self and identity. Being available means having the time and interest to listen to and observe the problems children face and being able to help them come up with solutions.

As stated above, we learn by trial and error, and no one needs to have ready-made solutions to the problems presented. However, children need to know that the interest is there and that parents and family members will lend their brainpower to the problems at hand. Feeling listened to bolsters a child's sense of worth while the opposite occurs when being brushed aside and ignored. Helping children come up with their own answers enhances their sense of self most and prepares them for future self-reliance.

WILL WE ALWAYS SEE DANGER?

Just as the biological immune system is geared to detect dangerous microorganisms, the psychological immune system is geared to detect dangerous elements in the environment and to seek opportunities to avoid them. For this reason, the threats and dangers we face always take priority in our awareness. We are programmed to look for them. You become aroused when you hear a loud unfamiliar noise, squealing brakes, see a flash of light, feel something crawling on your skin, smell smoke within your home, or find your child coming home in tears. You become anxious when a letter or phone call relates to the the job you were seeking, the school you applied to or the contest you entered. These situations reach one's awareness in a hurry, and when they do, we react intuitively. Later however we draw up plans to deal with them based on our experience, knowledge, superstitions, and beliefs. So, although we are stuck with a protective system that scans the horizon for threats, danger and opportunities, we are not stuck with responses and plans that are encased in cement.

Although we humans have developed clothing to protect us against cold, shelters to protect us from the elements and wild animals, water and food resources to deal with our thirst and hunger, tools and machines to magnify our strength, medical procedures to deal with physical injuries and diseases, psychological treatments to deal with injuries to our sense of self and identity, and economic systems to regulate our financial transactions with others, we still rely on weapons to capture or kill beasts and men who are seen as dangerous or threatening. So humans in the twenty-first century will continue to create and use new weapons despite the fact that we already have enough lethal weapons to destroy mankind three times over. All it takes to kill another human being is the pull of a finger on a trigger. As can be seen from the case of the hunter who killed six others while deer hunting, the two teenage boys who gunned down their fellow students at Columbine High School or the widespread killings around the world, weapons will continue to be used, made more efficient and more lethal. The National Rifle Association keeps saying that the problem is not the weapons but the people who use them. I guess the logic of this argument seems to be that if we ban enough people from using guns there will be less killing. Perhaps the slogan should be "keep the weapons, but ban the people." Think about what all-powerful fantasies were realized when a person was given the means to eliminate someone else with the pull of a finger. With today's weapons, a finger-pull can wipe out, not one, but scores of people. As if there weren't enough weapons on earth, serious consideration is being given to put weapons in space.[4]

REAL THREATS, IMAGINED THREATS AND WHO KNOWS

As long as we're programmed to keep looking for threats and danger in the twenty- first century and beyond, whether on an individual, group, or national level, it is imperative that we have ways of distinguishing friend from foe, real threats and great danger from non-threats and little danger, and that we have the means and ability to act on those distinctions. If such distinctions can't be made or are ignored, we're in for a lot of trouble, and the consequences could be grave.

Parents worry about this all the time, and in a society as complex as ours parents have the difficult task of trying to provide rules and admonitions to keep their children safe. When my colleagues, Dr. Kris Eisenhart and Sally Newell, and I presented a sexual abuse prevention program to elementary school children we asked them what rules their parents told them to follow when going to and from school, when playing outside, when home alone, and if they get lost.

Some of the answers we got were as follows: (1) always walk with a friend or friends going to or from school; (2) never get into a car with strangers; (3) don't talk to strangers; (4) look both ways before crossing the street; (5) don't run after a ball if it rolls into the street; (6) lock the door if you're home alone; (7) don't answer the door if you don't know who it is; (8) if someone calls, tell them your mother or father is in the bathroom and can't come to the phone right now; (9) if you're lost look for a policeman or a grownup taking care of a store; (10) know your address and phone number so someone can call your home if your hurt or lost; (11) if someone you don't know grabs you, scream, yell loud, kick them, and run.

From the rules these children mentioned it is clear that parents worry about them being abducted or abused by strangers, struck by automobiles, and having sufficient knowledge to handle being lost or injured. Thus, their antennae is focused on immediate type threats to their children's life and physical well-being.

Parents do make some rules about property and possessions, and sometimes about children standing up for their dignity. For example, nobody has the right to take your stuff without your permission, and nobody has the right to make fun of you and treat you unfairly. But the primary focus of parents is on the life and physical well-being of their children. They probably figure that if a threat is not immediate then they could get involved and handle the situation. Children, of course, have their own set of rules to live by, gathered from their own experience or that of their peers, such as which part of town is dangerous to walk in, which kids to stay away from, which kids not to antagonize because of their temper, and what not to do in school, around adults, and in public places. Against these of course, there's the excitement of doing something risky, egged on by the awareness that one's peers are sitting in judgment, and the need to show others that they will not "chicken out."

As children get older and are more influenced by their peers, the gap between what parents and children think are dangerous activities can be quite wide. It can be pretty scary for parents when their kids learn to drive and get their own cars. Parents say, "Now be careful" and kids say "Okay, okay, I've heard that already! Don't worry so much." The principles of the psychological immune system say that parents will continue to worry about their children until they're on their own because that's what parents are programmed to do, and parents evaluate their own sense of self on their ability to protect their children and have them grow into independent adults.

Wouldn't it be nice if kids said "Thanks for worrying about me" instead of, "Stop being such a worry wart." But age-influenced perspective is always an important factor in selecting what to worry about. And among a group of people, there are certainly individual differences. What's a threat to one person may not be a threat to another. It is known, in fact, that how easily and how quickly fear is produced depends on one's genetic predisposition and the scary situations or traumas they have experienced. [5, 6] This means that some people who see a dog running loose will immediately be apprehensive, while others will not react until they determine how friendly the dog is; that some people will be more frightened of the dark than others; and some people will anticipate disaster more rapidly than others when their cars break down on a lonely stretch of highway. Culture and superstition also play their parts in seeing threats and danger to oneself or others, and often prescribe ways to avoid or eliminate the danger.

For instance, according to Leo Igwe, head of the Nigerian Skeptics Society in Africa, most Nigerians believe in the existence of supernatural beings and believe these beings can be influenced through ritual acts and sacrifice. In addition, many Nigerians believe in ghosts, *juju* (the magic power of amulets), charms, and witchcraft that can protect individuals against business failures, sickness and diseases, accidents, and spiritual attacks. Many of the magical potions depend on the use of body parts, and as a result hundreds of kidnappings, ritual killings, and mutilations take place every year.[7] This is a stark example of how imagined threats and false beliefs can have a radical effect on other human beings. False beliefs go hand in hand with the fear generated by judging others according to skin color, ethnic identity or religious affiliation. This, too, carries the potential of disastrous results.

People now have access to all parts of the world through communication media like newspapers, magazines, radio, television, cell phones, and the Internet. These media compete for existence in a free-market, profit-oriented economy. Over the years publishers and advertisers have learned what grabs the public's interest. That's why the public is bombarded by reports of accidents, murders, kidnappings, rapes, robberies, home invasions, and sexual molestation. As a result, the public is led to believe that such things occur much more frequently and much closer to home than they actually do. Our natural vigilance for threats and danger is enhanced by this media blitz, and a background of fear pervades everyday life. Unfortunately, this sets the background for leaders and government to take advantage of us when they have agendas to pursue. A great example was the continual fear-mongering about the weapons of mass destruction in Iraq and that country's connection to Al Qaeda, even though none existed. Fear-generating statements, if repeated long enough by our leaders, can become part of our belief system, and once they take hold they are difficult to get rid of.

This was made clear to me when I was in the army and stationed in Germany ten years after the Second World War. I was working in a medical clinic, giving immunization shots. Also working in the clinic, assisting the army doctors, was a very intelligent German nurse who was married to an American with a Ph.D. in philosophy. We talked frequently about anything and everything. I was quite impressed by the broad knowledge she had of the medical community and how people interact with each other. One day she spouted out some stereotypical views of Jews being lazy. I was startled, to say the least, and I asked her where she had gotten her views. She stated, "That's what Hitler said!" Despite Hitler's defeat, the exposure of Nazi lies and cruelty in the Nuremberg trials, and the subhuman beliefs that were the basis for Hitler's genocidal policies, this nurse still hung on to the propaganda she had heard ten years earlier, her intelligence notwithstanding. This was a pretty scary example of the lasting effects of propaganda from leaders on high. Can we expect to see less reporting of murder and mayhem by the media or less use of propaganda by governments in the twenty-first century? It doesn't look that way.

HOW PROPERTY AND POSSESSIONS FIT IN

A tenet of the psychological immune system is that protection, preservation and/or enhancement of property and possessions is built into our makeup. How we value our property and possessions depends on what use we make of them and what meaning we assign to them. They can be things that protect us, things that make us more attractive, tools we make use of, creations of our imagination, or things collected as a hobby. The more value we put on them, the more carefully we protect them. Possessions can also take on symbolic value, become status symbols, or develop spiritual significance.

Weapons can take on symbolic value. In Yemen, for example, a country just south of Saudi Arabia, almost every home in this country of 17 million has at least one firearm. Guns are part of Yemeni culture, and owning them is a symbol of status and manhood. In some rural areas students even take their guns to school. Many tribal leaders have arsenals including mortars, machine guns, and rocket launchers.

Children learn to use weapons as early as ten years of age, and it becomes a hobby and a sport. Former Prime Minister Abdul-Karim al-Iriani said in an interview, "Yemenis have possessed arms since the first rifle was invented in the world. Yemenis have never been disarmed, so we know it's not possible to do it unless there's a total economic and social change in the country to make the possession of arms irrelevant." Some estimates have maintained that there are three weapons for every person in the country.[8]

In South Africa, property in the form of land has deep spiritual and cultural significance. Pride and dignity go with the ownership of land. As a field worker told a correspondent, "You need land in order to be recognized in Africa. Without land you are nothing." While political power and economic prosperity are very important to South Africans, what seems to matter most is their spiritual and cultural connection to the soil that holds the graves of their forefathers.[9]

In America, the term "pride of ownership" is heard especially in regard to homes; but this usually takes second place to the dollar value that land or houses have. On the other hand, some Indian tribes look at land as something more than its monetary value. For example, Margie Mejia, tribal chairwoman of the Lytton Band of Pomo Indians in Sonoma County, stated, "Land represents something sacred to Indians. Without land of your own, there's no place to practice your culture. You become nothing but a stepchild, a black sheep." Unfortunately, this tiny band of Indians is landless, but they are trying to buy fifty acres in a wooded region about fifty miles north of San Francisco.[10]

In the twenty-first century, property and possessions will continue to play an important part in the lives of practically everyone whether for practical reasons, monetary ones or symbolic ones. However, there are differences of opinion about what should or should not be considered property. If you own something you consider it your property. In this way of thinking, then, domestic dogs, cats and horses are property. Some people, however, think of their pets as part of their families and take exception to the notion that pets can be equated with other forms of property like radios, dishwashers, vacuum cleaners, and coin collections. If monetary value is the deciding factor, how about comparing pets to computers, cars, houses, and bank accounts? Many people would still maintain that live animals cannot be defined as property, just as live people cannot.

This, however, has not always been the case. In the infamous 1857 Dred Scott decision, the U.S. Supreme Court ruled that a slave was not a person but property and therefore Congress could not forbid slavery in the territories without violating a slaveowner's constitutional right to own property. It wasn't until after the Civil War that slaves were given citizenship and civil rights with the adoption of the Fourteenth Amendment in 1868.[11]

While the question of whether a person can legally be considered property is no longer an issue, the question of whether living organisms and life's processes are property or products that can be owned, was among the issues being wrestled with in the twentieth century, and continues to be debated today. If an individual or corporation can claim ownership of something invented or created, like a new drug or new medical device, it can apply for a patent. If the patent is granted, then anyone using the product can be required to pay a user fee. The owner has a right to rent, sell, or make other arrangements for his patent and the right lasts for twenty years in the United States. Patenting living things like genes, genetically modified animals, and medicines from plants has become a contentious issue.

The problem of patenting living things reared its ugly head in 1971 when the U.S. Patent and Trademark Office (PTO) rejected a patent request from an Indian microbiologist working for General Electric for a genetically engineered bacterium that could consume oil spills. They stated that living things are not patentable under U.S. patent law. However, in 1980 the U.S. Supreme Court overruled the PTO and determined, for the first time, that a patent, could be given on a genetically engineered life form. Then, in 1987, the PTO issued a ruling that all genetically engineered multicellular living organisms, including animals, were open to being patented. This represented a complete about-face from its 1971 ruling.

In fact, the PTO granted a patent on the first mammal, a genetically engineered mouse. Since then, patents have been applied for on nearly 200 genetically modified animals including pigs, cows, and sheep. These animals are used to study cancer and other diseases by inserting genes that were not originally part of the animals. This has led to the discussion of finding mutated genes in humans and inserting new or modified genes to correct potential anomalies like Down syndrome, spina bifida, Tay-Sachs disease, and sickle-cell anemia. Likewise, worldwide searches are under way for new patentable "discoveries" that many native peoples claim have already been discovered by them and are being pirated by large corporations. An example is curare, an important surgical anesthetic and muscle relaxant derived from plant extracts, that has been used by Amazonian Indians for generations to stun prey.[12]

So it seems that living things, other than humans, can be classified as property and owned by individuals, corporations, and governments. They can be patented if they have been modified in some way that allows them to be used as an aid to human activity. Genetic engineering and modifications of plants and animals will continue to be important for scientific and commercial purposes in the twenty-first century with predictable objections from indigenous people and organizations like the Council for Responsible Genetics, who would like to draft legislation to exclude living organisms and their parts from the patent system, including human genes.[13] The last updated guidelines from the U.S. Patent and Trademark Office reaffirmed that companies may patent both whole genes and pieces of genes as long as they can establish a particular use for them. The PTO asserts that since a gene may be removed from a person and a clone of that gene may be made by a machine, which is not part of nature, the gene is a product of the lab. Therefore it can be considered someone's property and can be patented if its use can be shown.[14]

However, a debate is still going on about what to call animals that have human genes or human stem cells inserted into them which have the potential of making organs with human cells and human function. What happens to a sheep with human brain cells; is it still a sheep, or a man in sheep's clothing? The debate brings out the question of how far we can and should go in altering life forms if we are uncertain about the outcome? The question seems to touch on both science and ethics and it's a question that people will struggle with in the twenty-first century.

As the above presentation shows, property and possessions play an important role in human society and reinforce the contention of the psychological immune system that there is a built-in predisposition to protect, preserve and enhance our property and possessions. This fits with what I overheard a mother say to her three-year old daughter: "No matter how much I buy for you it is never enough; you always want more!" This statement is music to the ears of the advertising industry, which works hard to perpetuate the urge to buy more. It also reflects the creativity of children and adults, who use their imaginations to envision new and more varied products, and provides the foundation for the creation of intellectual property, which is taking on a greater and greater role in the economic life of the country. As Armen A. Alchian, an emeritus professor of economics at UCLA maintains, "the purported conflict between property rights and human rights is a mirage-property rights are human rights."[15]

SENSE OF SELF AND IDENTITY IN THE 21ST CENTURY

The first thing a mother hears from a doctor or nurse, when her baby is born, is : "Mrs. Jones, you have a girl," or "Mrs. Jones, you have a boy." If the baby looks fine then the word "healthy" may be inserted before "boy" or "girl." Assigning a sexual identity to a child seems to be a significant first step for the parents in the process of overseeing and guiding the development of the child's sense of self and identity. It provides a foundation for interaction with their child. Parents know what clothes and toys to buy, and what to anticipate telling their friends and relatives, who are surely going to ask whether they had a girl or boy.

The psychological immune system, as conceived, maintains that humans are programmed to protect, preserve and/or enhance their own sense of self and identity as it develops and matures. It also maintains that parents are programmed to protect, preserve, and/or enhance the sense of self and identity of their children. And, in fact, many parents judge their own worth and identity by how well they are doing in helping their children learn about and adapt to the day-to-day world they live in. So, if the doctor tells the parents about a problem with their newborn child, that may affect the child's self image and makes recommendations to correct or eliminate the problem, the parents will more than likely follow the advice of the doctor even if surgery is recommended. This scenario comes up frequently when children are born with ambiguous genitals and questionable sexual identities resulting from gene mutations that affect the hormonal output of the adrenal glands.

As a parent, what would you do if your obstetrician told you that your newborn child was most likely a girl but had no vaginal opening and an enlarged clitoris that could be mistaken for a penis? Or, suppose the physician said your child was most likely a boy, but showed no testicles and had a micropenis that looked more like a clitoris. The doctor states that with surgery the genitals could be made to look more normal, so that in later years your child wouldn't have to face living with deformed sexual parts and endure the shame and humiliation that comes with this condition and they will know their sexual identity for sure. What parent wouldn't want to correct faulty sexual parts and make sure their child knew what his or her gender was as they grew up? The whole issue seems to belong to the medical profession, which has diagnosed and offered surgical treatment for the problem of "intersexed" children.

But caution should be exercised when the suggestion is made that an individual's self image or sense of self can be made whole or enhanced mainly or solely through medical procedures, especially if the individual is not in a position to consent to those procedures. Corrective surgery for ambiguous sexual parts falls into this category since the decision is made not by the child but by the parents at the prompting of the medical staff involved.

In fact, an organization was founded in 1993 called The Intersex Society of North America (ISNA) which is "devoted to systematic change to end shame, secrecy, and unwanted genital surgeries for people born with an anatomy that someone decided is not standard for male or female." The society was founded by Cheryl Chase, who was herself diagnosed as an intersex child and who underwent genital surgery that left her scarred and unable to experience orgasm. The Society has offered guiding tips for parents such as getting in touch with a psychologist, psychiatrist, or social worker "who has experience dealing with gender issues and birth anomalies." It notes that "caring medical doctors-including endocrinologists, urologists, and surgeons-may try to provide counseling to you and your child on the fly, but most have neither the time nor training to do it well." ISNA cautions that surgical reconstruction may leave a child with diminished sexual sensation, scarring, and a poor cosmetic outcome, and that many parents have raised children with sexual ambiguity who are grateful for their parents' decision not to have surgery. The society maintains that waiting until the child is old enough-at least a teenager-to decide whether to have cosmetic genital surgery supports an individual's right to make decisions affecting his or her identity.[16, 17] The society currently has many professionally qualified physicians, psychiatrists and psychologists on its medical advisory board.

An individual's sense of self is certainly tied up with his or her sexual identity and how well he or she fits in with and is accepted by his or her peers. But, sexual identity or gender acceptance depends on more than external genitals. There are individuals with normal male genitals who feel more like females and some even opt to undergo radical surgery and take hormone injections to convert themselves to women. Conversely, there are individuals with normal female genitalia who feel they have the disposition of males and want to convert their bodies into male bodies and opt for surgery and hormone injections to accomplish their goals.

Some, like Dr. Renee Richards, a popular tennis player and physician who was surgically converted from male to female, later regretted the decision. Richards felt "not as fulfilled (as a woman) as I dreamed of being."[18] Others, however, have been satisfied with their decisions to surgically change their sexual identities because emotionally they had already identified with the gender they eventually converted to. The point is that sexual identity is a complex condition that includes a genetic foundation, the way the genes express themselves, the impact of the environment and social milieu on the expression of one's genetic makeup, and an individual's acceptance of what he or she looks like, feels like, and how he or she is treated by others. Body parts do not make up one's identity, just as one's identity does not make up one's body parts. The more that individuals have the freedom to determine how they want to look and be, the more likely they are to accept the end results. Children who have no say so in how they are surgically transformed are much more likely to reject the transformation when they become older and more self-aware. So parents who, with the best of intentions, opt to rely on surgery to correct the ambiguous genitals their children could be born with, may want to wait until their children are old enough to determine their own sexual identity.

The case of David Reimer is a vivid example of what can develop when a child too young to be a willing participant undergoes surgery to change his gender.

The facts of the case presented below are based on two accounts. One was written by John Calapinto in 1997 for the *Rolling Stone* magazine who, with the Reimer family's consent, was given access to family interviews about what transpired during the thirty years since David Reimer's surgery was performed.[19] The other was written by David Usborne in 2004 for Reality Resources,[20] based on his research into the case.

The original surgery took place as the result of a strong recommendation by Dr. John Money, a research psychologist at Johns Hopkins Medical Center, who was considered an expert on human sexuality, sexual identity problems, and children born with ambiguous genitals. Dr. Money made the recommendation to David's mother to have David undergo surgery to reassign him as a female after he learned that David's penis had been accidentally "burned off" by a cauterizing instrument during circumcision. Since David's mother was desperate to help her son and Dr. Money was considered the exert in the field, she took his recommendation to give David a sex-change operation, change his name, and raise him as a female. Dr. Money's research on the influence of genetics and culture - or nature versus nurture - on sexual identity convinced him that if a child underwent a sex change operation before thirty months of age and was raised as surgery dictated, the child would take on and accept that sexual identity. This would happen, he stated, as long as the parents reacted to the child as though the new gender was the normal one.

Dr. Money considered this case a particularly relevant test of his theoretical outlook on the role culture plays in determining sexual identity because David was surgically reassigned within the thirty-month period and he happened to have an identical twin brother whose circumcision had come out normal. Thus Dr. Money could keep track of how sexual identity developed in identical twins, one raised as a boy and the other raised as a girl. The case generated a considerable amount of interest in the scientific community, and Dr. Money was willing to feed the demand for information through his lectures and his writing. He kept in touch with David's mother on a regular basis. Their conversations and her letters seemed to confirm that David was adjusting well to his female identity and was much different from his twin brother. Dr. Money's continual pronouncements of how successfully things were going prompted a write-up in *Time* magazine in 1973, and his book, *Man, Woman, Boy, Girl,* was praised by *The New York Times Book Review.* One child psychologist at Johns Hopkins related that the undisputed success of the twins experiment legitimized the practice of infant sex reassignment globally.

However, what Dr. Money didn't anticipate or check for was that the progress related to him by David's mother was colored by her vested interest in seeing her son adjust well to his new gender so that she didn't have to wrestle with the possibility of having made the wrong decision. John Colapinto's interviews with the twins underscored the biased reporting the mother gave to Dr. Money. For example, David's twin brother related that when they were in grade one or two he "saw all the other girls doing their thing-combing their hair, holding their dolls." His sister (David), however, "was not like that. Not at all." She expressed an ambition to be a garbage man. "She'd say, 'Easy job, good pay.'" He recalled, "She was six or seven years old. I thought it was kinda bizarre - my sister a garbage man?" When he told his mother about his sister's behavior, she would tell him that his sister was being a "tomboy." He told Colapinto, "I recognized Joan (David's pseudonym) as my sister, but she never, ever acted the part. She'd get a skipping rope for a gift, and the only thing we'd use that for was to tie people up, whip people with it. Never used it for what it was bought for."

David never seemed comfortable with his gender, even though he didn't learn about what had happened to him until he was thirteen years old. He rejected Dr. Money's urging to undergo additional vaginal surgery at age eight and stated that he daydreamed about being a twenty-one-year-old male with a mustache and a sports car. His supervising psychiatrist, Dr. Keith Sigmundson, noted that the experiment was falling apart by the time David was eleven years old. When David's father finally explained what had happened to him when he was a child, David immediately demanded surgery and hormone treatments to change him back to a male. His parents complied and this surgery was completed when he was sixteen years of age. This entailed having his breasts removed and an artificial penis constructed (which however was not capable of erection). His relationships with girls created much anxiety, and when at age eighteen, he entrusted his secret to a sixteen-year-old girl he was dating, he quickly became the object of muttered comments, giggles, and ridicule from his peers. He made a suicide attempt and was found unconscious by his parents, but was taken to a hospital in time and recovered.

After his brother married and became a father, David was quite envious and stated that this was everything he had wanted to do since high school. The brother and his wife introduced David to a young woman with three children who was three years his senior. They hit it off and David married her at age twenty-five. He eventually adopted the children. After David's story was published in *Rolling Stone* and he appeared on the

Oprah Winfrey show, his anguish was opened to the whole world. For reasons that have never been made clear, David's brother took his own life in 2002, which hit David very hard. Then his wife left him, taking the children with her, and David became very depressed. In May 2004, at the age of thirty-eight, he also ended up taking his own life - a tragic ending to the story of a boy rebelling against the attempt to impose an identity on him that he couldn't accept.[20]

As this story shows, an important part of the job of individuals in protecting, preserving, and/or enhancing their sense of self and identity is clarifying and evaluating who they are, which may be at odds with the way others define them or want them to be. This job of clarification and evaluation is a never-ending process, maintained by the psychological immune system, just as the protection of the body by the biological immune system is never-ending. So, battling against forces that want to shape one's identity and sense of self, even though well intentioned, can be a lifetime struggle.

Sometime back, homosexuality was seen as a psychiatric disorder or mental illness, and many states passed laws against homosexual activity. This view was vehemently challenged by homosexuals and they were finally removed from the mentally ill category. Nevertheless, the fight to elevate their status to that of heterosexuals continues to meet with resistance in the twenty-first century because there are social forces that feel threatened, especially on religious grounds. So, having overcome its identity as mentally ill, the homosexual community now must overcome its identity as morally ill.

As a member of a family and society, there are certain standards and roles that everyone is expected to adopt and adhere to. When these boundaries are challenged, breached, or believed to be breached, the family and society feel their authority is under attack, and pressure is applied to push the offending member or members back into the accepted boundaries. Family and social pressure can be quite daunting, and individuals who are uncomfortable with the standards and roles imposed on them will tend to seek out others who share their discomfort. This is a protective strategy that can produce confrontations with other social forces. Accusations and issues of right and wrong are then fought out in the public arena such as gay marriage, the use of marihuana for medical purposes, polygamy, violent video games and punishment or rehabilitation for law violators.

Wards at the California Youth Authority, many of whom were victims of abusive families or who were taken advantage of by adults when they were children, talked about principles they used to prevent the hurt that comes from trusting people and being let down. Many of the same principles were also used by abused, neglected, and rejected children to create a state of mind to protect them against further injury to their sense of self.

Here are some of those principles: 1) Don't try if you don't have to, you'll only fail again; 2) Don't get your hopes built up, they'll only get dashed again; 3) Don't expect fair treatment, you'll only end up disappointed again; 4) Don't let people know how much you need them, you'll only end up getting hurt again; 5) Don't listen to what people say, they'll only change their mind later on and confuse you more; 6) Don't trust people, you'll only get let down again; 7) Don't act weak or scared, you'll only get stepped on and used; 8) Do unto others before they do unto you; 9) Tune your emotions out; keep them hidden. They'll only cause problems for you; 10) There's on rhyme nor reason to the world; trying to find one just creates more confusion.

In a competitive world where one has to deal with cycles of disappointment, frustration, and failure, followed by surprise, smooth sailing, and success, it certainly helps to develop mindsets and principles that protect against injury to one's sense of self and identity on the down cycles. How successful people are in doing so may determine their ability to avoid deep depression and emotional impairment. "Always think positively and expect success" and "If things can go wrong, they will," are two such different mindsets.

CONTROLLING THE PSYCHOLOGICAL IMMUNE SYSTEM

Since environmental and social forces can be powerful instigators and the psychological immune system can produce powerful responses, there have to be ways of preventing overreaction. The speed and intensity of a reaction by the psychological immune system depend on the amount of fear generated and the degree of emotional hurt experienced. The greater the fear and the greater the emotional hurt, the greater the speed and intensity of a reaction.

As pointed out previously, the prefrontal cortex has the job of preventing inappropriate responses that are prompted by the amygdala, the emotional center of the brain. The prefrontal cortex monitors an individual's performance so that corrections and adjustments can be made as the reactions proceed. This process can be observed pretty clearly when you are driving down the road and someone decides to cut in front of you with little or no notification. You are startled, and your psychological immune system is strongly activated by the threat of bodily harm to yourself and your passengers, the threat of damage to your vehicle, and the insult to your sense of self and identity. You hit the brakes, blow the horn and experience a rush of emotion. You blurt out (out-loud or under your breath) a barrage of cuss words and shout "why don't you watch where you're going? Who the do you think you are, anyway?" Then you get the impulse to retaliate. You want to ram the violator's vehicle, cut back in front of him or her, and yell out your window with a gesture that indicates your displeasure. These emotional urges and outbursts are filtered through your prefrontal cortex, and what emerges are the actions you take. You are doing what is known as "weighing your options."

This process happens very rapidly, and your final reactions are based on a number of considerations: whether you sense that your life and physical well-being will be more jeopardized by retaliating or letting the other driver know of your displeasure; whether you anticipate that retaliating could lead to damage to your vehicle, and whether you see yourself as a person who knows better than to act irrationally or impulsively. These considerations also generate emotional responses, which may come out as fantasies of what you would like to do. These emotions and fantasies can compete with your original emotional responses and urges. If you feel obsessively challenged by the other driver, or if you feel that nobody has the right to put you in jeopardy this way, and if these feelings cannot be contained, then you are likely to retaliate in some way. This kind of "road rage" can lead to violent acts, sometimes even death.

Keeping the psychological immune system in check is no easy matter once it is triggered by threats to one's life or physical well-being, one's property and possessions or one's sense of self and identity. Under most circumstances it functions like the biological immune system,which is regulated by a homeostatic mechanism, that is, it is activated, remains activated until it meets the challenges confronting it, and then falls back to a normal, non-threatened level. If the intensity of the psychological immune system is not damped but remains active for too long, it can lead to both psychological and neurological damage.

The strength and lethality of the psychological immune system can be inferred from the widespread killings of people in the twentieth century who were considered threats to each other or their governments. Excluding killings that occurred during wartime, some 60 to 70 million people were killed in ethnic, tribal, and government- sponsored acts. If wars are included, the figure goes up to 80 or 90 million people. As asserted by a doctor from Yugoslavia who saw and heard killings going on day and night, "In any man, in any human being, we have one uncontrolled monstrous animal. This animal is suppressed, by culture, by education, by religion. And if you have power in your hands, and if you have newspapers and radios and television and you are prepared to awaken this animal, you can be very successful."[21]

THE IMPACT OF FAIRNESS, JUSTICE AND EQUALITY ON THE PSYCHOLOGICAL IMMUNE SYSTEM

It has been pretty well established that chimpanzees react with a kind of moralistic aggression when a member of their troop does not reciprocate in kind to other chimps who have helped it.[22] This type of behavior seems to be a precursor to the human tendency to evaluate the behavior of others as "just" or "unjust" and react with anger to unjust behavior.[23] As pointed out in Chapter III, the development of a standard for behavior, a sort of moral compass, allowed human groups to become vast in size compared to the chimpanzees, who have to rely on a leader and his coalition to control other troop members. Thus, sexual behavior in the presence of the leader with a female the leader favors, is met with aggression from the leader. In early humans, sexual behavior could be regulated by the family and the community using a moral compass to determine what was an acceptable standard and what was not. The leader, in the form of a warlord, nobleman, king, prime minister or president, didn't have to be present as long as everyone was on the same wavelength regarding the behavior standards. This applied to other areas of behavior, as well, such as interpersonal conflict, property rights, and demeaning one's neighbors.

The development of moral and ethical standards for human behavior has been a major factor in controlling the innate or instinctual urge of the psychological immune system to neutralize, eliminate, or destroy whatever is considered a threat to one's life, property, or identity. This is one of the filters used by our prefrontal cortex, our evaluative center, in controlling the impulsive urges and preventing inappropriate responses directed by our emotional center, the amygdala.

The moral stance has been effective on many occasions, as when used by such leaders as Martin Luther King Jr., Nelson Mandela, and Mahatma Gandhi to stop violence by the state against its own members. Unfortunately, there have been more instances of violence being reinforced by taking a "moral" stance. In such cases the argument is that "they are breaking the rules, upsetting social order, violating laws or are a threat to the government, so they must and will be stopped." When morality sanctions the innate impulse of the psychological immune system, its lethality can be legend. The 90 million people killed in the twentieth century and the millions already killed in the twenty-first century are a testimonial to this proposition. It's a formula for unrestrained killing since it is declared as protecting, preserving, and enhancing, the physical well-being and the identity of the state and loyal citizens.

Throughout human history, codes of conduct have been used to either create institutions of justice or to justify genocide and wars. In the final analysis, the dependence of human beings on force-to enforce court orders, break up fights, keep demonstrations within bounds, protect the public against criminals, and root out terrorists and keep the homeland safe from "evil" nations-assures the humans race that those who have the most power and the biggest muscles will end up ruling and will determine from their perspective what is moral, just and fair.

The creation of the Universal Declaration of Human Rights by the United Nations, which will be sixty years old in 2008, was a noble effort to produce a universal code of conduct for all nations to follow. But while nations may talk universally, they act nationally and look out for their own physical well-being, property and possessions and identity, which is translated into reputation and influence. It is difficult for nations-or any groups-to maintain their concern for others when any of the components of their psychological immune systems is perceived to be under threat. The same principle holds true for the individual and the family. You protect yourself and your family first, before you help other people and other families. Exception are rare.

THE DANCE OF LIFE

If the 4.5 billion years since the earth was formed were condensed into a twelve- month period, life would have begun in

February, apes would have evolved in late December, and modern humans would have appeared on December 31 minutes before midnight. We have not been here that long, and like all animals before us we are fighting for our existence. We have been given great gifts. We can use symbols and create symbolic systems such as mathematics, language and science; we can plan ahead; we can pretend, use simulators, and role-play; we can represent our visions, thoughts, and feelings in artistic form; and we can create societies that encompass millions of people and thousands of rules and regulations to define what is acceptable and not acceptable. But the question remains, has evolution dealt us a losing hand?

Evolution has given us a biological immune system that helps defend the body against pathogens that could do us harm. This system relies almost entirely on its ability to detect and identify cells that belong to the person it protects and cells that do not. Without this ability it wouldn't have a clue when to spring into action. But while evolution has given us this protective system, it has also provided many microorganisms the means to create novel strategies to evade detection. As a leading immunologist stated, "The variety and ingenuity of these escape mechanisms are most intriguing and, as with virtually all infectious agents, if you can think of a possible avoidance strategy, some microbe will already have used it."[24] So, the dance of life continues between the microbes that are trying to escape the wrath of the biological immune system and the defenses created by the system.

Now the psychological immune system has come along, programmed to protect, preserve. and enhance human life and physical well-being by alerting people to danger and providing the urgency and means to deal with them. Microbes that have been able to evade the defenses of the biological immune system have produced infections and diseases. This has activated the psychological immune system's emotional response of fear, created a sense of urgency and mobized energy to deal with these threats to human life. Initially, humans prayed to heavenly forces and spirits for relief, and some people still rely on spiritual healing, but over decades, the medical and pharmaceutical industries have been created to carry out this protective imperative of the psychological immune system. Through study and scientific experimentation humans have been able to better understand how to deal with disease and lend a hand to the biological immune system. So the dance of life continues between human ingenuity to deal with the microbes that evade the defenses of the biological immune system and the evolved ability of the microbes to resist and overcome our medical and pharmaceutical strategies.

In many ways, the psychological immune system, uses the same defensive mechanisms as the biological immune system. One of its main purposes is also to detect and identify threats to one's life and physical well-being. Microbes and diseases can be detected and identified; but how about humans who are threats to other humans? How about detecting and identifying "terrorists" and others who want harm to certain groups, countries or individuals. This has become a major problem in the twenty-first century and has led to the creation of a super intelligence agency in the United States, The Department of Homeland Security, and legislation like the Patriot Act, which gives the police and intelligence agencies greater power to investigate and surveil, even compromising the rights of citizens to be secure in their private lives. The argument is that the mandate to provide safety and security in a time of peril trumps everything else, including many human rights. So, now we have the "good" humans trying to detect and identify the "bad" humans. One group uses detection technology, and the other group uses evasive technology, and the dance goes on.

For better or for worse, the psychological immune system has also been programmed to protect, preserve, and enhance our sense of self and identity. The variety of cultures, ethnic groups, and social backgrounds, as well as the variables provided by status, socioeconomic standing, and exposure to hardship, makes the sense of self and identity of humans a very rich, complex, and varied conceptual entity. How does one go about trying to protect all these different components, and how does a society go about trying to protect, preserve, and enhance the sense of self and identity of its members? Have any industries developed, like the medical and pharmaceutical ones, to deal with threats to people's sense of self and identity? Is this the job of the mental health community or human right groups? Is there a consensus in the world that there are effective procedures and organizations to deal with injury and trauma to people's sense of self and identity? How are threats, injuries, and trauma to one's sense of self and identity related to the list of mental illnesses in the latest *Diagnostic and Statistical*

Manual (DSM IV)? Some disorders such as Post Traumatic Stress Disorder and Acute Stress Disorder, do deal with intense psychological distress that is caused by exposure to traumatic events, but injury to one's sense of self and identity is only inferred but not specified.

My experience with trauma victims-most of whom have experienced physical or sexual abuse-has left me with the strong impression that they are forever wrestling with questions pertaining to their sense of self and identity. "Am I partially to blame?" "Could I have done anything differently?" "Why did I act like I did?" "I wonder what other people think of me?" How do I get over my self-disgust?" and " What will I do if the same situation occurs again?" are some of the questions that keep coming up. Some of the principles to develop a protective state of mind have already been given Yet, their outrage and rage permeate their state of being when memories of the abuse emerge-and they emerge frequently. Many go on, despite the traumatic experiences, to lead productive lives and maintain a healthy sense of self and identity. So how exactly related are injury to one's sense of self and identity and mental illness remains unclear and is complicated by the complex influences of various cultures on the foundation and ongoing construction of one's identity and the various experiences that produce changes in and to one's sense of self.

Perhaps it can be argued that a universal method of protecting, preserving, and enhancing the human sense of self and identity would be to provide a social structure where humans of all ages could learn how to perform tasks in a way that gives them a strong sense of accomplishment. This would provide them with a sense of worth, self-esteem and a well-defined sense of self that could withstand most threats and injuries. But what if one group's sense of accomplishment is based on beating out or outdoing another group? Then injury to the identity of the second group would lead to the need to retaliate, and a cycle of trouble would develop. How about a sense of accomplishment based on killing the members of another group who are considered threats? We can all comprehend the cycle of death and destruction that this would create. Unfortunately, this state of affairs has been and still is all too common.

It seems as though our sense of self and identity is the highlight of being human and the glue that binds us to one another. Just as our cells maintain and are nourished by the makeup of the body, our identity maintains and is nourished by the makeup of the group. Yet it causes us the most difficulty because it has the potential to pit one person against another and one group against another. The psychological immune system is programmed to be a protective system, and as such it directs us to look for the threats to ourselves, our families and our nation. So we keep trying to detect and identify "non-self" members so that we can keep "self" members safe. Our technology keeps getting more sophisticated and our methods of detection more widespread, even using the satellites circling the earth. But sophisticated technology and methods of evasion are not granted to only one group of people. We all have the same brainpower and planning abilities.

So, the game of life goes on, which unfortunately includes the game of death. If we don't learn that the psychological immune system has the same lethal potential as the biological immune system and ways to keep it under control we are in for more and more destruction. Our best hope is a global realization of this fact and the urgency to see each other as self-members. We have to keep our lethality in check using our knowledge and planning. The United Nations has made an attempt to do this with some success. We need a United Nations made up of children from all the nations who learn to see each other as members of a large family. This would give humanity some hope of not wasting the wonderful gifts of evolution.

CHAPTER I
References

1. Demasio, A. R. (1994) *Descarte's Error,* New York: Avon Books.

2. Nesse, R. M. and Williams, G. C. (1994) *Why We Get Sick : The New Science of Darwinian Medicine,* New York: Vintage.

3. Rifkin, J. (1998) *The Biotech Century.* New York: Jeremy P. Tarcher/ Putnam.

4. Fredrickson, J. K. and T. C. Onstott (1996) Microbes Deep Inside The Earth, *Scientific American,* 275, no 4, p. 68-71.

5. Kerr, R. A. (1997) Life Goes to Extremes in the Deep Earth-and Elsewhere?, *Science* 276, no 5313, p.703.

6. Oliwenstein, L. (1995) Death and the Microbe, *Discover* 16, no 9, p 98-103.

7. Ibid. 103

8. Breakthroughs (1995) The Epiphyte's Friend, *Discover* 16, no 8, p 16.

9. Nesse and Williams *Why Sick,* p. 78-84 (see 2. above)

10. Breakthroughs: (1996) Baked Hornet Japonais, *Discover* 17, no 2, p. 16.

11. MacQuitty, M. (1995) *Megabugs : The Natural History Museum of Insects ,* L. Mound, Scientific Advisor, New York: Barnes and Noble.

12. Frank, A. (1997) Quantum Honeybees, *Discover* 18, no 18, p. 80-87.

13. L.M. Tierney Jr, S.J. McPhee, and M.A.Papadakis, eds. (1996) *Medical Diagnosis and Treatment,* 35th ed. Stanford: Appelton and Lange, Chaps 31-34

14. Roitt, I. M. (1994) *Essential Immunology,* 8th ed. Cambridge: Blackwell Scientific Publications.

15. Audesirk, G. and T. Audesirk (1989) *Biology: Life on Earth,* 2nd ed. New York: Macmillian.

16. Roitt (1994) *Immunology,* Chap 12 (see 14. above)

17. Price, S. A. and L. M. Wilson, eds. (1986) *Pathophysiology: Clinical Concepts of Disease Processes ,* 3rd ed. New York: McGraw-Hill.

18. Roitt (1994) *Immunology,* Chap 2 (see 14. above)

19. Parijs, L.V. and Abbas, A.K. (1998) Homeostasis and Self-Tolerance in the Immune System: Turning Lymphocytes Off, *Science*, 280, no 5361, p. 243-248.

20. Sopolsky, R. M. (1996) Why Stress Is Bad for Your Brain, *Science*, 273, no 5276 p. 749-750.

21. Abrams, G. D. (1986) Response of the Body to Immunological Challenge, *Pathophysiology* , Price, S.A. and L.M. Wilson, eds. New York: Mcgraw-Hill, p.68.

22. Adelman, D. C. and Terr, A. (1997) Allergic and Immunologic Disorders in *Medical Diagnosis and Treatment* (1997), p. 724-749 (see 13. above)

23. Roitt (1994) *Immunology,* Chap 19 and 20 (see 14 above)

24. Whitcare, C. C., et al. (1999) A Gender Gap in Autoimmunity, Science, 283, no 5406 p. 1277-1278.

25. Estes, R. D. (1991) *The Behavior Guide to African Mammals,* Los Angeles: The University of California Press, p. 449-456.

26. Johanson, D. and Edgar, B. (1996) *From Lucy to Language,* New York: Simon and Shuster.

27. Ibid. p 88

28. Price, D, H. (1990) *Atlas of World Cultures,* Newbury Park, Calif.: Sage Publications.

29. Caird, R. (1994) *Ape Man:The Story of Human Evolution,* New York: Macmillan.

30. Leakey, R. (1994) *The Origin of Humankind,* New York: Basic Books.

31. Johanson and Edgar (1996) *Lucy to Language,* p. 96-97 (see 26. above)

32. Cousins, N. (1979) *Anatomy of an Illness,* New York: W. W. Norton and Co.

33. Duin, N. and Sutcliffe, J. (1992) *A History of Medicine,* New York: Barnes and Noble.

34. Caird (1994) *Ape Man,* p. 147 (see 29. above)

35. Davidson, I. and Noble, W. (1995) When Did Language Begin?, *The First Humans: The Illustrated History of Humankind,* American Museum of Natural History, G. Burenhult, ed. New York: Harper Collins, p. 46-53.

36. Duin and Sutcliffe (1992) *History Of Medicine,* p. 14 (see 33. above)

37. Ibid. p. 16

38.Cartwright, F. F. (1972) *Disease and History,* New York: Dorset Press

39. Ibid. p 46

40. Richardson, S. (1995) The Return of The Plague, *Discover,* 16, no 1, p. 69.

41. Marshall, E. (1996) The Genome Program's Conscience, *Science,* 274, no 5287 p. 488-490.

42. Pennisi, E. (2003) Human Genome: Reaching Their Goal Early, Sequencing Labs Celebrate, *Science* 300, no 5618, p. 409.

CHAPTER II
References

1. Einstein, A. (1954) Chicago Address, Decalogue Society, *The Great Quotations*, G. Seldes, ed. (1972) New York: Pocket Books.

2. Bach, M. (1961) *Strange Sects and Curious Cults*, New York: Dorset Press.

3. Hernandez, R E (1995) Proud of being stupid, *Ventura County Star*, 9 June.

4. Rosato, J. Jr. (1996) Simi High Nails 5th-Place Finish at Academic Decathlon, *Ventura County Star*, 11 March.

5. The name of the High School has been omitted from the article

6. The name of the coach has been omitted from the article

7. Bentley, A. (1994) Police Laud Man as "Hero," *Ventura County Star*, 22 September.

8. The Associated Press (1994) Boys Slaying Strikes at Italy's Soul, *Ventura County Star* 1 October.

9. Weatherford, J. (1994) *Savages and Civilization*, New York: Crown Publishers, Inc.

10. Weiss, P. (1980) Idiocide, *Evaluation and Change*, special issue, Program Evaluation Resource Center, Minneapolis Medical Research Foundation, Inc.

11. Legal Information Institute (1996) *Bennis v Michigan*, (94-8729), 517 U.S. 1163, Tina B. Bennis, petitioner v Michigan, on Writ of Certiorari to the Supreme Court of Michigan, March 4, 1996, Legal Information Institute.

12. Amnesty International (1995) *Amnesty Action*, Summer, New York: Amnesty International USA.

13. Koestler, A. (1974) The Limits of Man and His Predicament, *The Limits Of Human Nature*, J. Benthall, ed. New York: E.P. Dutton & Co.

14. Amnesty International (1995) *Amnesty Action*, Spring, New York: Amnesty International USA.

15. The Associated Press (1994) Massacre in Rwanda, *Ventura County Star*, 16 May.

16. E. Bobley and R. Bobley, eds. (1977) *Illustrated World Encyclopedia,* Woodbury, New York: Bobley Publishing Co. p 458.

17. Timmerman, K. (1994) Suicide Bomber, *Response :The Wiesenthal Center World Report*, vol 15, no 3, Fall/Winter, 1994/95, p2

CHAPTER III
References   *75A*

1. Danzer, R. (1993) *The Psychosomatic Delusion,* New York: The Free Press.

2. Russell, R. J. (1993) *The Lemur's Legacy,* New York: G.P. Putnam's Sons.

3. Goodall, J. (1990) *Through a Window: My Thirty Years with the Chimpanzees of Gombe,* Boston: Houghton Mifflin Co.

4. Garraty J. A., and P. Gay, eds. (1972) *The Columbia History of the World,* New York: Harper & Row, p. 61.

5. De Waal, F.B.M. (1992) The Chimpanzee's Sense of Social Justice and Its Relation to the Human Sense of Justice, *The Sense of Justice,* R. D. Masters, and M. Gruter, eds. Newbury Park: Sage Publications.

6. Leakey, R (1994) *The Origin of Humankind,* New York: Basic Books.

7. Caird, R. (1994) *Ape Man: The Story of Human Evolution,* New York: Macmillan.

8. Shreeve, J. (1996) Sunset on the Savanna, *Discover,* 17, no 7, p. 116-125.

9. Weatherford, J. (1994) *Savages and Civilization,* New York: Crown.

CHAPTER IV
References

1. LeDoux, J. (1996) *The Emotional Brain: The Mysterious Underpinnings of Emotional Life,* New York: Simon & Shuster.

2. Demasio, A. R. (1994) *Decarte's Error,* New York: Avon Books,

3. LeDoux, J. (1996) *Emotional Brain* p. 203-205. (see 1. above)

4. Farb, P. (1986) *Man's Rise to Civilization,* New York: Avon Books p. 85-86.

5. B. Goran, ed. (1995) *The First Humans : Human Origins and History to 10,000 BC.* American Museum Of Natural History, San Francisco: Harper.

6. J.A.Garraty and P. Gay, eds. (1981) *The Columbia History of the World,* New York: Dorset Press.

7. Estes, R. D. (1991) *The Behavior Guide to African Mammals,* Berkley and Los Angeles: The University of California Press.

8. Goodall, J. (1990) *Through a Window: My Thirty Year With The Chimpanzees of Gombe,* Boston: Houghton Mifflin Co.

9. Stevens, W. K., (1999) *Gabon Logging Pushes Chimps into Deadly Wars,* Ventura County Star, 18 May.

10. Schultz, J. L. (1999) *Why Dogs Bite, Animal Watch,* (ASPCA), Summer, p. 24.

11. J.A. Garraty and P. Gay, (1981) _Columbia History_, p. 59 (see 6. above)

12. Amnesty International (1994) _Amnesty International Report 1994,_ New York: Amnesty International Publications.

13. Amnesty International (1998) _Amnesty International Report 1998,_ New York: Amnesty International Publications.

14. Clifton, T. and S. Mazumdar, (1999) _The War In Thin Air,_ Newsweek, 12 July, p. 35.

15. Bellisle, M. (1999) _Activist Ignores Death Warnings,_ Associated Press, Ventura County Star. 11 March.

16. Zimbardo, P. G. (1992) _Psychology and Life,_ 13th ed. New York: Harper Collins p. 600.

17. Nathanson, D. (1992) _Shame and Pride: Affect, Sex, and the Birth of the Self,_ New York: W.W. Norton and Co.

18. Farb, P. (1986) _Man's Rise_ , p. 66-68. (see 4. above)

19. Ibid, p 135

CHAPTER V
References

1. Zimbardo, P. G. (1992) *Psychology and Life,* 13th ed. New York: Harper Collins.

2. Asimov, I. (1989) *Asimov's Chronology of Science and Discovery* , New York: Harper & Row, pg. 5.

3. Greenspan, S. and Greenspan, N. I. (1985) *First Feelings : Milestones in the Emotional Development of Your Baby and Child,* New York: Viking Penguin Inc.

4. Kagan, J. (1994) *The Nature of the Child*, 10th ed. New York: Basic Books.

5. Brim, O. G. and J. Kagan, eds. (1980) *Constancy And Change In Human Development*, Cambridge: Harvard University Press.

6. Reitman, V. (2002) Two Days of Torment, Triumph, *Los Angeles Times*, 1 Jan.

7. Farb, P. (1968) *Man's Rise To Civilization*, New York: Avon Books, p.38.

8. Ibid

9. Walker, A. and Parmar, P. (1993) *Warrior Marks*, New York: Harcourt Brace & Co, p.38.

10. Johanson, D. and Blake, E. (1996) *From Lucy To Language*, New York: Simon & Shuster.

11. Jung, C. G., ed. (1964) *Man and his Symbols*, New York: Doubleday & Company, Inc.

12. Locke, M. (2002) Her Life Feels Like the Center of a Tornado, The Associated Press, *Ventura County Star*, 11 June.

13. Lajoie, R. (2001) Courage of the Morning, *Amnesty Now*, winter 2001-2002, New York: Amnesty International USA, p.12.

14. Harris, B. (2005) Aung San Suu Kyi: Hero File, *Moreorless*, June 2005. www. moreorless.au.com/heroes/suukyi.html

15. Associated Press (2003) SuuKyi Home After Surgery, but Still Held, *Los Angeles Times*, 27 September.

16. Balasundaram, F. J., ed. (1997) Martyrs in the History of Christianity, Indian Society for Promoting Christian Knowledge, Delhi, India. (prepared for "Religion Online," by Ted and Winnie Brock)

17. *Western Inquirer* (1999) Los Angeles: Center for Scientific Investigation of Claims of the Paranormal (CSICOP), Mar.-Apr. 1999.

18. Moveni, A. and S. Rotella (2003) Iranian Jurist Wins Nobel Peace Prize, *Los Angeles Times*, 11 October.

19. Koehler, T. (1998) Murder-Suicide Called Act of Love, *Ventura County Star*, 8 Nov.

20. Eisenberger, N. I., Lieberman, M. D., and Williams, K. D. (2003) Does Rejection Hurt? An fMRI Study of Social Exclusion, *Science,* 302, no 5643, p.290.

21. Irons, P. and Guitton, S. (1993) *May It Please The Court : The Most Significant Oral Arguments Made Before The Supreme Court Since 1955,* New York: The New Press.

22. Rosenblatt, R. (1991) The Bill of Rights : The First of the 10 Amendments Launches Us on a Journey of Self-Discovery, *Life,* Bicentennial Issue, Fall Special, 1991

23. Rotstein, A. H. (2000) Six Illegal Immigrants Die of Exposure in Past Week, Associated Press, *Ventura County Star,* 6 June.

24. Associated Press, (2000) Brothers Die After Fall Into Icy Pond, *Ventura County Star,* 22 Dec.

25. Jamison, L. (2003) Killing For 'Honor,' Legalized Murder, *Amnesty Now,* Amnesty International USA, Vol 29, Summer 2003.

26. Scripps Howard News Service, (1999) Love Match Might Be Fatal, *Ventuta County Star,* 2 Jan.

27. Dixon, R. (2001) Adoption Brings Joy To One Family, Pain To Another, *Los Angeles Times,* 18 Feb.

28. Siegel, D. J. (1999) *The Developing Mind* , New York: Guilford Press.

CHAPTER VI
References

1. Evans I. (1998) Ghosttowns: Eldoradoville, Phoenix: Atjeu Publishing LLC (2004) www.ghosttowns.com/states/ca/eloradoville.html

2. Steele, B. (1998) Ghosttowns: Zurich, Phoenix: Atjeu Publishing LLC (2004) www.ghosttowns.com/states/ca/zurich.html

3. McCurnin, T and Grumbo, J. (1998) Ghosttowns: Canyon Diablo, Phoenix: Atjeu Publishing LLC (2004) www. ghosttowns.com/ states/az/canyondiablo.html

4. Ghosttowns.com (1998) Ghosttowns: Greaterville, Phoenix: Atjeu Publishing LLC (2004) www. ghosttowns.com/states/az/ greaterville.html

5. Bleifuss, J. (1998) Know Thine Enemy: A Brief History of Corporations, *These Times*, Feb. www.thirdworldtraveler.com/Corporations/KnowEnemy- Itt.html

6. Lasn, K. (1999) *Culture Jam: The Uncooling of America*, New York: William Morrow and Company.

7. Glasberg, D. S. and Skidmore, D. (1998) The Dialectics of White - Collar Crime: The Anatomy of the Savings and Loan Crisis and the Case of Silverado Banking, Savings and Loan Association-Special Invited Issue: Money, Trust, Speculation and Social Justice-Part 1: Trust, Confidence, and Crime, *American Journal of Economics Sociology* , Oct. 1998.

8. Jameson, R. (2002) Case study: US Savings and Loan Crisis, *ERisk Report*, Aug. 2002.

9. Simon, H. A. (1997) *Administrative Behavior*, 4th ed. New York: The Free Press.

10. Leeming, D. A. (1990) *The World of Myth*, New York: Oxford University Press

11. Weatherford, J. (1994) *Savages And Civilization: Who Will Survive?*, New York: Crown Publishers, Inc.,

12. *Encyclopaedia Britannica, Ready Reference 2003* CD-ROM, Chicago: Encyclopaedia Britannica Inc., (2002)

13. Ibid

14. Siegel, D. J. (1999) *The Developing Mind: Toward a Neurobiology of Interpersonal Experience*, New York: The Guilford Press.

15. Kagan, J. (1994) *The Nature of the Child*, Tenth anniversary edition, New York: Basic Books

16. Taylor, M. (1996) From Two Worlds, in *Where Masks Still Dance : New Guinea*, by C. Rainer (1996) New York: Little Brown & Co.

17. Zinn, H. (1995) *A People's History of the United States 1492 - Present*, New York: Harper Perennial.

18. Worster, D. (1979) *Dust Bowl: The Southern Plains in the 1930s*, New York: Oxford University Press.

19. Peltz, J. F. (2004) Kroger Sets Aside Funds for Rivals, *Los Angeles Times*, 20 April.

20. Vieth, W. and La Ganga, M (2004) _Firms Often Avoided Taxes, Los Angeles Times_, 7 April.

21. Britannica Ready Reference (see 12. above)

22. Paddock, R. C.(2002) The Crime of Being a Young Refugee, _Los Angeles Times_, 5 January

23. Associated Press (1997) Sterilization Stirs Anger, _Ventura County Star_, 19 December

24. United States Holocaust Memorial Museum. Handicapped, Washington, D.C.: United States Holocaust Memorial Museum

25. Satsuk, I, (1999) The Children of the Camps Project, _National Asian Telecommunications Association_, www. children-of-the-camps.org

26. Zinn (1995) A People's History, p. 407-408 (see 17. above)

27. Wertman,V. F. (2003) Righteous Gentiles Among Nations: A Selected Annotated Bibliography, _MultiCultural Review_, December.

28. United States Holocaust Memorial Museum. Jehovah's Witnesses: Victims of the Nazi Era, 1933-1945, Washington, D.C.: United States Holocaust Memorial Museum

29. Cozzens, L. (1997) The Civil Rights Movement 1955-1965: Birmingham, http://www.watson.org/~lisa/blackhistory/civil rights-55-65/selma.html

30. Marahaj, D. (2004) When the Push for Survival Is a Full Time Job, _Los Angeles Times_, 11 July.

31. Perry, T. (2002) A Voice Suddenly Heard, *Los Angeles Times Magazine*, 7 July.

32. Miller, L. and France, D. et al. (2002) Sins of the Fathers: The Catholic Church Confronts Shameful Secrets, *Newsweek*, 4 March.

33. Guccione, J. (2004) Subpoena of Church Records Rejected, *Los Angeles Times*, 14 July.

34. Mehren, E. (2004) A Parish and Its Faithful, in Limbo, *Los Angeles Times*, 9 July

35. General Motors Corporation (2004) GM and Focus: Hope, Partners for a Better Future. www.gm.com/company

36. Ford Motor Company (2004) Overview : Our Vision, Our Mission, Our Values.www.ford.com/en/company

37. Nader, R. (1965) *Unsafe at Any Speed :The Designed-in Dangers of the American Automobile*, New York: Grossman Publishers.

38. Nader, R. (1959) The Safe Car You Can't Buy, *The Nation*, 11 April.

39. Bollier, D. (1989) Citizen Action and Other Big Ideas: A History of Ralph Nader and the Modern Consumer Movement, Washington, D.C. : Center for the Study of Responsive Law.

40. The Center for Auto Safety (2004) Ford Pinto Fuel-Fed Fires, Washington, D.C., The Center for Auto Safety, 2004. www.autosafety.org/article.php?scid=145&did=522

41. Ellis, M. (2004) Suzuki Drops Lawsuit vs. Consumer Reports, Reuters, *The Washington Post*, 8 July. www.WashingtonPost.com

42. Guest, J. (2004) Truth and consequences: *Suzuki vs. Consumers Union, Consumer Reports*, "Have You Heard," department, March. 172D

43. Kennedy, M J. (2002) Return of the Warrior: Truth and Consequences on the Reservation, *Los Angeles Times Magazine*, 7 July.

44. *Indian Trust.* (2004) Cobell v. Norton, 7 July. www.indiantrust. com,

45 The People's Republic of China (2004) Constitution Of The People's Republic of China (adopted December 4, 1982, updated March 22, 2004) *People's Daily Online* July 2, 2005. english.people.com.on/ constitution/constitution.html

46. Wong, B. (2004) China and the Internet, New York: Internet Communications, 1 August. www. bobsonwong.com/research/china

47. Zittrain, J. and Edelman, B. (2002) Empirical Analysis of Internet Filtering in China, *Berkman Center for Internet & Society*, Harvard Law School, November.

48. Banisar, D. (2003) The Great Firewall of China, *Amnesty Now*, Spring, vol XXIX, No 1, New York: Amnesty International USA.

49. United Nations (2000-2005) Human Rights: Fiftieth Anniversary of the Universal Declaration of Human Rights 1948-1998, United Nations 2005. www.un.org/Overview/rights.html

50. United Nations (1987) Fact Sheet No. 4; Methods of Combating Torture, Office of the High Commissioner for Human Rights, Geneva, Switzerland, December 1987. www.unhchr.ch/html/menu 6/2/fs4.html

51. Human Rights Web (1997) A Summary of United Nations Agreements on Human Rights, 8 July 1994. www.hrweb.org/legal/ undocs.html

52. Amnesty International (1999) Amnesty International Report 1999 Documents a Rise in Violations, *Amnesty Action*, Amnesty International USA, Summer 1999

53. Serrano, R. A. (2004) Pentagon Cites Widespread Involvement in Prison Abuses, *Los Angeles Times*, 26 August

CHAPTER VII
References

1. LeDoux, J. (1996) *The Emotional Brain: The Mysterious Underpinnings of Emotional Life,* New York: Simon & Shuster.

2. Ridderinkhoff, R K. et al. (2004) The Role of the Medial Frontal Cortex in Cognitive Control, *Science ,* 306, no 5695, p. 443-446.

3. Audesirk, G and Audesirk, T. (1980) *Biology: Life on Earth*, 2nd ed. New York: Macmillan Publishing Co. p. 284.

4. Leonard, D. (2005) Weapons in Space: Dawn of a New Era, Space. com., 17 June, Nuclear Policy Research Institute. www. nuclearpolicy.org

5. Bourne, E. J. (1990) *The Anxiety & Phobia Workbook,* Oakland: New Harbinger Publications, Inc.

6. Hariri, A. R. et al. (2002) Serotonin Transporter Genetic Variation and the Response of the Human Amygdala, *Science*, 297, no 5580, p. 400-403.

7. Igwe, L. (2004) Ritual Killings and Pseudoscience in Nigeria, *Skeptical Briefs*, Newsletter of the Committee for the Scientific Investigation of Claims of the Paranormal, 14, no 2, June.

8. Abu-Nasr, D. (2000) Arsenals a Manly Art in Yemen, The Associated Press, *Ventura County Star ,* 23 March.

9. Simmons, A.M. (2003) A Hunger for Land of Ancestors, *Los Angeles Times*, 17 January.

10. Glionna, J. M. (2002) Community, Landless Tribe in Dispute, *Los Angeles Times*, 18 March.

11. World Book Multimedia Encyclopedia (2001) Dred Scott Decision, Mac OS X Edition, Version 6.0.2, Chicago: World Book, Inc.

12. Rifkin, J. (1998) *The Biotech Century*, New York: Jeremy P. Tarcher/Putnam.

13. Charnas, R. (2002) "No Patents on Life" Working Group Update, *Genewatch*, 15, no 3, May-June, Council for Responsible Genetics, 2004. www.gene-watch.org/genewatch/articles/15-3update.html 207B

14. American Medical Association, (2004) Gene Patent Guidelines, *AMA Science*, 9 November. www. ama-assn.org/ama/pub/category/print/3607.html

15. Alchian, A. A. (1993) Property Rights, *The Concise Encyclopedia of Economics* Library of Economics and Liberty. www. econlib. org/library/Enc/Property Rights.html

16. Intersex Society of North America-ISNA (2004) A World Free of Shame, Secrecy, and Unwanted Genital Surgery, ISNA 1993-2004. www.isna.org

17. Intersex Society of North America-ISNA (2004) Guiding Tips for Parents, ISNA 1993-2005. www.isna.org/node/63

18. *Reality Resources* (2004) Dr. Renee Richards, Lexington: Reality Resources Publications. www.realityresources.com/drreneerichards.htm

19. Colapinto, J. (1997) The True Story of John/Joan, *Rolling Stone*, 11 December, InfoCircHome, 2004. http://infocirc.org/rollston.htm

20. Usborne, D. (2004) Tragic End of David Reimer, *Reality Resources*, 12 May, Lexington: Reality Resources Publications. www.realityresources.com/tragic.htm

21. Levinson, A. (1995) Genocide a Thriving Doctrine in the 20th century, The Associated Press, *Ventura County Star,* 18 September.

22. De Waal, F.B.M. (1992) The Chimpanzee's Sense of Social Regularity and Its Relation to the Human Sense of Justice, *The Sense of Justice: Biological Foundation of Law*, Masters, R. D and M. Gruter, eds. Newbury Park: Sage Publications.

23. McGuire, M. T. (1992) Moralistic Aggression, Processing Mechanisms, and the Brain, *The Sense of Justice: Biological Foundation of Law*, Masters, R.D. and M.Gruter, eds. Newbury Park: Sage Publications

24. Roitt, I. (1994) *Essential Immunology*, 8th ed. Cambridge: Blackwell Scientific Publications.

About the Author

Dr. Kagan has been a licensed practicing clinical child psychologist for well over thirty years and found the time to write this book only because he finally retired. He is hopeful that the information in the book will eventually be helpful to his grandchildren when they become adults. He received his Ph.D. in clinical psychology from the University of Arizona and has worked for a private psychiatric hospital, the California Youth Authority and the County of Ventura. He has extensive experience with abused children and their families and has taught many courses for the University of California, Santa Barbara Extension program.

www.ingramcontent.com/pod-product-compliance
Lightning Source LLC
Chambersburg PA
CBHW031826170526
45157CB00001B/194